LIVING WITHOUT A HEART BEAT

STEVEN JACOBS

ISBN: 978-1-953865-81-6 (Paperback)
ISBN: 978-1-953865-82-3 (eBook)
Lorenzo: Translation from Dutch to English, proofreader
Caro Geeraerts: Illustrations
Library of Congress Control Number: 2024915343
Books Fluent
New Orleans, Louisana

CONTENTS

PREFACE   V

INTRODUCTION   IX

CHAPTER 1:   THE HEART AND HOW IT
                 FUNCTIONS   3

CHAPTER 2:   DISEASES OF OUR HEART   27

CHAPTER 3:   TREATMENT OF ACUTE AND
                 CHRONIC HEART FAILURE   49

CHAPTER 4:   MECHANICAL HEART PUMPS   63

CHAPTER 5:   HEART PUMP IMPLANTATION   83

CHAPTER 6:   LIVING WITH A HEART PUMP   133

CHAPTER 7:   DANGERS OF LIVING WITH A
                 HEART PUMP   151

CHAPTER 8:   A LOOK AT OUR LVAD PROGRAM   169

CHAPTER 9:   THE FUTURE OF HEART PUMPS   177

CHAPTER 10: END OF LIFE WITH A
                 HEART PUMP   189

EPILOGUE   197

PREFACE

MICHAEL IS A FIFTY-SIX-YEAR-OLD, HAPPILY MARRIED business owner. He's tough as nails—a hard worker and a bit of an overachiever. He loves his family, and he loves a good game of golf with his close friends. Today, he's happily hitting a few golf balls and enjoying a truly wonderful day. Life is amazing!

This day, however, will be tragically different. It all starts with a painful pressing sensation in his chest—something that he never felt before. Michael sits down to catch a breath, yet the pain has no plans to subside. He's beginning to grow weary and frightened—something very serious and dangerous is unfolding right in front of his eyes. Before anyone can notice Michael's deteriorating condition, he suddenly loses consciousness and collapses on the ground. The bystanders start administering CPR (cardiopulmonary resuscitation) and notify the emergency services as Michael's day rapidly descends into a living nightmare.

Michael has just suffered a massive myocardial infarction, commonly known as a *heart attack*. The blood vessels that surround his heart and provide the needed oxygen to the body's engine have shut down completely. As Michael's heart is starved of oxygen, it ceases to function entirely. Just a few agonizing seconds later, as the brain is desperately gasping for fresh oxygen, Michael loses consciousness. His life hangs by a thread.

Thirty nerve-racking minutes later, the emergency physicians fail to restart his heart and decide to transfer him to the hospital. As the ambulance is skillfully negotiating the narrow Belgian streets, the emergency crew notifies the emergency room staff. The short ambulance ride seems to stretch for an eternity . . . Inside the hospital, the staff prepares everything, ready to rescue another life as the crucial seconds slip away.

As Michael arrives, he is put directly onto the operating table. The surgeons skillfully make an incision in the groin to find direct access into the large blood vessels and connect the entire cardiovascular system to a machine. This machine now becomes Michael's heart and lungs. The blood flows through one tube directly into the device, where the blood is enriched with oxygen, pressurized, and sent back to the body—providing every organ with fresh oxygen in the process. For now, Michael's body and brain will have a chance to recover from this tragic event. Today, he looked straight into the cold, empty eyes of death and was lucky to survive.

Just one and a half hours into the tragedy, Michael's life has been saved. However, the blood vessels to his heart are still obstructed and need to be addressed immediately. The specialists from the cardiac catheterization unit try their best to free the blocked heart vessels, but to no avail. The damage is simply too severe.

Still unconscious, Michael is transferred to the intensive care unit, where he slowly recovers and starts showing signs of improvement. His kidneys, liver, and lungs are slowly recovering from the traumatic, life-threatening event that took place on the golf course. Michael eventually wakes up and finally processes the severity of his current reality. The bad news is he's still connected to the machine that provides his body with oxygenated blood. He has been chained to his hospital bed for the past five days, and his heart still fails to function properly on its own. The good news—he's alive! This machine is a true modern miracle. Thanks to the tireless efforts of the surgeons and the reliability of the artificial heart-lung machine, Michael is literally given a second chance at life.

One week after the tragic events, Michael enters the operation room for the second time. The surgeons remove the tubes connected to the blood vessels in his groin and attach a small device directly to his heart. Compared to the bulky machine that kept him alive for seven days, this device is tiny—no bigger than a clenched fist. In the medical world, this small machine is called an LVAD (left ventricular assist device).

It literally takes over the function of the heart and allows the blood to circulate around the body.

This tiny pump is implanted in Michael's chest. Only a small, thin cable that serves as a power supply exits the body near his abdomen. The operation is a success! Now Michael needs two more weeks to make a full recovery and learn about the intricacies of the LVAD.

After the two weeks pass, Michael is finally free to return home and rediscover his second life. Walking, working, and even playing golf are now again possible thanks to the amazing small pump that lives in his chest. Aside from a battery pack and small computer, he doesn't need any other bulky devices that would hinder his daily activities. The only strange feeling that he's not used to is his complete lack of a heartbeat. When he touches his wrist, there's no pulse! The machine is doing all the hard work in the background, with a light, monotonous buzzing sound emanating from his chest. The buzzing sound comes from a propeller spinning at 5,000 rpm inside the LVAD and pushing the blood to his organs at a constant rate of five liters per minute.

Six months after the myocardial infarction, Michael is deemed a good candidate for a heart transplant. He now must wait for a suitable donor heart to appear. After almost two years of Zen-like patience, Michael's turn finally comes to receives his long-awaited heart transplant.

Luckily for Michael, his story has a happy ending. Every single year, thousands of people around the world are saved by the amazing LVAD as the heart becomes too weak to circulate blood around the body. Michael's story is 100 percent real. It is just one of the many ways that patients with a failing heart end up with an LVAD. As we continue, we will discuss many other interesting examples from my professional experience.

INTRODUCTION

FOR HUNDREDS OF YEARS THE HUMAN HEART WAS CON-
sidered inoperable. This amazing biological engine that drives our
body—constantly in motion—was simply beyond the realm of possibilities for surgeons from the pages of our history books. You may not
know this, but during the Middle Ages, the masters of surgical craft
were already successfully performing amputations and even removed
bladder stones. Yet, medical science had to wait until September 9, 1896,
to witness the very first heart surgery.

In Frankfurt, Germany, Ludwig Rehn had saved the life of a twenty-two-year-old man by stitching a wound found on his heart. The
subsequent publication of Rehn's work awarded him well-deserved
fame and recognition in the medical field, as well as opened the door
to an entirely new medical practice—heart surgery.

As the developments in the medical field continued, it took well into
1925 to see surgeries performed on the inside of the human heart—
mainly on the valves. In those early days, the surgeon broke calcifica-
tions on the heart valve using only his finger. This allowed stenotic
valves to open better. The procedure was performed via a small incision
on the side of the heart and had to be done quickly to prevent serious
blood loss. The moment the valve was free from obstructions, the surgeon closed the incision.

Although we were finally able to work on the human heart, it was
still vital that the heart kept beating during these surgeries to provide
the body and brain with enough blood to survive the operation. We
couldn't lose too much blood either. Needless to say, surgeons back
then were working with their backs against the wall. After WW2, new

solutions were developed and subsequently helped to propel the art of heart surgery even further. For example, children with hereditary heart defects were put under anesthesia and placed into an ice bath—reducing the body temperature to below 20 degrees Celsius (68 degrees Fahrenheit). At this temperature, the heart stops beating, and the body's oxygen and general energy use are almost at a standstill. This allowed the surgeons time to operate without having to worry about the beating of the heart or critical blood loss.

Of course, manipulating the body temperature is quite risky for the patient; hence, we went out searching for a way to circulate blood around the body without the need for the heart itself as the engine of blood circulation. One clever solution was connecting the blood circulatory system of the child to one of the parents. This method was effective; however, a completely autonomous "artificial" heart would be a much better solution. The heart-lung machines made their debut during the 1950s, and for the first time in medical history, it was possible not only to circulate blood without the need for a human heart but also to enrich it with oxygen in the process—a true medical revolution in heart surgery. Working on a human heart became safer and more straightforward than ever before.

These amazing machines taught us an important lesson: It doesn't really matter *how* the blood circulates inside our body—with the help of the heart itself or by machine. As long as the blood is enriched with oxygen and this blood circulates across all blood vessels, your body will always function perfectly!

Our heart is a wonderful yet very simple organ. In essence, it is no more than an engine pushing fluids through tubes. Our kidneys clean our blood, our liver breaks down harmful substances, and our pancreas regulates our glucose levels (no matter if you subscribe to a strict diet or gobble up an entire chocolate cake in one sitting). All these activities involve complex chemical processes at molecular, even atomic levels. But what about our heart? Our heart simply pumps blood and circulates it around our body, beat after beat after beat. No fancy chemistry going on here (except maybe when you fall in love). Of course, it's not all as simple as it looks. The heart's electrical impulses must be administered at precise intervals just to function properly. A plethora of hormones and nerve impulses play together to manage muscle contractions. But if we put these technical factors aside for a moment, it's safe to conclude that our heart is simply an extremely reliable pump that circulates between four and twenty liters of blood across our body every single minute.

In the 1960s, engineers started playing around with these concepts and letting their minds run wild with questions such as: *What if your heart is too ill to work properly?* or *Wouldn't it be amazing to replace the heart with a pump that circulates blood, giving you decades of care-free life in the process?*

Back in the 1960s this sounded like a plot of a thrilling sci-fi movie, but today, this has become our reality. Every single year, thousands of people receive an artificial heart pump that helps—or replaces—the function of a weakened heart.

My name is Steven. I happen to be one of the people who performs these life-saving surgical procedures. I love what I do, and this book is the result of many years of passionate work. Together we will lift the veil of medical mystery and discover in a simple, fun, and entertaining way what these heart pumps are, what they can do, and what they may do for you or your loved ones someday. This book focuses on *left ventricular assist devices* (LVADs), which are heart pumps that assist the heart in circulating blood throughout the body. The devices that totally replace the heart (*total artificial hearts* or TAHs) are briefly mentioned but go beyond the scope of this book.

It took me two decades of med school, surgical internships, writing a thesis, attending tons of scientific meetings, and treating heart failure patients to build the knowledge I have today. In this book, I try to bring some of that knowledge to you without asking you to study medicine and become a doctor yourself. Inevitably this means that we cannot elaborate on every topic down to the last detail or cover all exceptions or treatment options. This book will give you a good understanding of heart failure and how mechanical heart pumps fit into the treatment of this disease, but not at a specialist level. So before we proceed, let's keep in mind that this is by no means a book about a possible treatment for your specific condition. Every one of us is different. Every patient's life path is unique and requires a partnership between you and your physician.

This book is also based on my experiences as a cardiac surgeon in Belgium. Every country has different ways of organizing healthcare and different demographics, and this leads to differences in our daily practice. Every cardiac surgery department makes its own protocols for the treatment and follow-up of patients. So don't be surprised if your hospital experiences were different from what you read here. Many roads lead to Rome! Or in this case, your healthy life with an LVAD.

This book is dedicated to all the people who work with LVAD patients, from the professor doing the operation to the nurse coming to the home of the patient to check the wound dressings. Treating patients is teamwork, and every contribution counts to ensure a good outcome.

I hope you have as much fun reading these words as I had writing them.

LIVING WITHOUT A HEART BEAT

CHAPTER 1

THE HEART AND HOW IT FUNCTIONS

WHEN WE PEEL AWAY THE COMPLEXITY, OUR HEART IS just a big muscle. All our muscles contract and relax—yet this muscle is quite unique. In fact, it's so unique that there's nothing in our body that even remotely resembles it. Think about it for a second: when your heart has to work flawlessly every second for the rest of your life, it better be special indeed!

Simple math illustrates this a lot better. Let's imagine that your heart beats just 60 times per minute. This adds up to 3,600 beats per hour, or 86,400 beats per day—for the rest of your life. Every year we cross a jaw-dropping 31 million beats, and if you really like to crunch numbers, you'll quickly arrive at a few billion heartbeats across an average human lifespan. In short, our heart is one amazingly reliable and efficient machine. It's okay to put the book down for a second and feel your own heartbeat as you take in these facts and numbers.

Our heart is literally built with flawless perfection in mind. It's a beautifully balanced orchestra of atriums, ventricles, nerves, and valves, synchronized to perfection—delivering oxygenated blood to our organs. If we look at other mammals and even birds, the design

Heart chambers

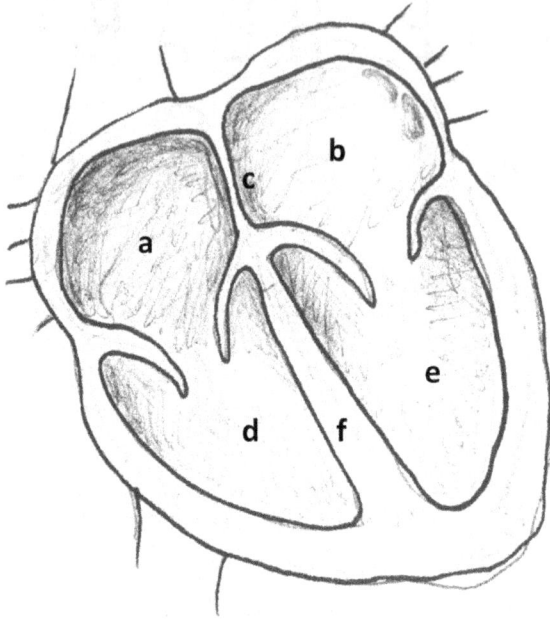

Figure 1.
In total there are four heart chambers. Two atriums (right atrium (a) and left atrium (b)) and two ventricles (right ventricle (d) and left ventricle (e)). Both atriums and ventricles are separated by a septum. The septum between the atriums is called the interatrial septum (c), the septum between the ventricles is the interventricular septum (f). The assembly of an atrium and ventricle works as a pump unit. So in fact our heart is composed of two pumps.

of their hearts looks very similar to our own. Evolution is a wonderful thing—you never need to change a winning team, and you don't go screwing around with an already perfect design.

Before we can dive into the main course of this book, it's important to establish some basic understanding of the anatomical and functional concepts. Not only will it be extremely interesting, but it will also give you a better understanding of how our heart actually works. Furthermore, it's pointless to explain the functions of implantable heart

Classic air pump

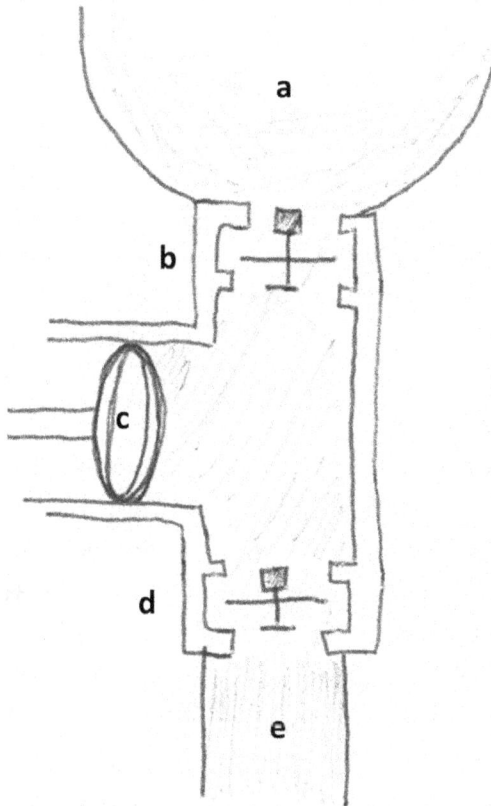

Figure 2.
The working of a classic air pump best resembles the working of our heart pump.
Air enters the pump through the inlet manifold (a). In our heart this would be the atrium.
A piston (c) compresses the air, creating pressure, and one-way valves (b and d) make sure the air only exits the pump at the outlet manifold (e). In our heart the piston motion is mimicked by the contracion of the ventricular wall. The one-way valves would be the atrio-ventricular (b) and semilunar valves (d).

pumps without first understanding the basics. Don't panic! This is not a complex medical course. We'll stick with the basics, and we'll have a blast learning all the interesting details using illustrations and simple examples. One thing I can guarantee you is that after this chapter, you'll be ready to dazzle your friends and colleagues with some awesome new knowledge. Let's dive right in.

ANATOMY OF THE HEART

Our heart is a hollow organ with walls that are pure muscle—a bit like your stomach but not quite the same. The inside of our heart is divided into four separate chambers that are filled with blood. There are two *atriums* and two *ventricles*. One atrium is always connected to one ventricle, and together they team up to form a single pump. If you think that four separate chambers should make two complete pumps, you would be 100 percent correct. In fact, our heart is a system of two separate pumps!

The blood arrives in the atrium and gets pumped away by the ventricle. Let's examine a classic air compressor that lives in the corner of your garage. The inlet manifold that is sucking in all the atmospheric air is the atrium. The heavy metal piston and cylinder assembly that's doing all the grunt work is the ventricle. Simple, right?

Our atriums don't need to work exceedingly hard—they have a rather thin layer of muscle. Remember how flimsy the inlet manifold of an air pump looks? It can even be made out of plastic or composite materials. When it comes to the ventricle, however, it's a completely different story. These chambers are more muscular and can handle extremely powerful and violent contractions. Again, let's think of the air compressor. The pistons and cylinder assembly are robust and heavy metal components that are doing all the huffing and puffing. They compress the air, get exceedingly hot in the process, and require quite a lot of cooling and lubrication. Our ventricles are, in essence, the same hard workers.

The easiest way to distinguish both heart pumps (atrium + ventricle assembly) is to look at their position in our body. One pair lies a bit more to the right and the other more to the left. Hence, we have the left and the right side. In summary, we have the left atrium and ventricle as well as the right atrium and ventricle. Pretty simple so far.

The right atrium and ventricle "assembly" provides blood only to the lungs. The left atrium and ventricle provide blood to our entire body. Although these two parts are built for different functions, they are inseparably connected inside one unit—the heart itself.

Naturally, all the parts are beautifully interconnected. Both the left and right atriums are located next to each other. The small part that divides the atriums is called a *septum*. If you guessed that there should be a septum between both ventricles, you are absolutely correct. It's called the *interventricular septum*. Remember that the left ventricle pumps the blood throughout our entire body, while the right one pumps only to our lungs? Naturally, that makes the left ventricle the absolute boss! It's bigger and stronger and provides a much more powerful contraction than its smaller brother on the right side.

The left ventricle muscle wall is thicker and much more robust. Even the shape of both ventricles is quite different. The small brother, the right ventricle, has a much more triangular shape, while the bigger brother, the left ventricle, is much rounder. The best way to remember the difference is to think of a deep-sea submersible. These vessels have a perfectly spherical shape that helps to withstand the monstrous pressure of deep-sea diving. More pressure means that a round shape is the best design for the left ventricle.

Now that you know about the atriums and ventricles, let's see what happens to the blood. After it visits the left side of the heart, it's pressurized and gets delivered to all our vital organs via a system of blood vessels that range from massive tube-like highways down to the smallest capillaries that are even smaller than a strand of your hair. During the pumping action, the flow of blood only happens in one direction! This is where valves enter the scene.

Our lives would be nothing without valves. Simply put, they ensure that the flow of liquid, air, and even gas goes in only one direction. The same happens inside our heart with the help of atrioventricular valves.

Bloodflow in the heart

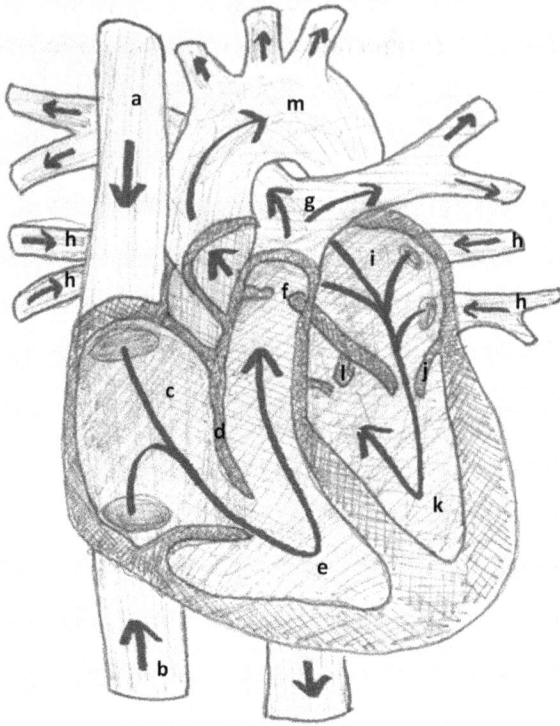

Figure 3.
Venous (deoxygenated) blood arrives in the right atrium (c) from the superior and inferior caval veins (a and b). It passes over the tricuspid vavle (d) into the right ventricle (e) from where it is pushed over the pulmonary valve (f) to the pulmonary artery (g) and further to the lungs. After receiving oxygen in the lungs the blood returns to the left atrium (i) through the four pulmonary veins (h). Oxygenated blood reaches the left ventricle (k) over the mitral valve (j) and is finally pushed to the aorta (m) over the aortic valve (l).

Don't be intimidated by the difficult-sounding medical lingo. The main principle is very simple: the valves prevent blood from flowing in the wrong direction. That's it!

If you really want to get into the nitty-gritty details, the right atrioventricular valve is called the *tricuspid valve*. The left one is called the *mitral valve*. Again, when the ventricles contract—creating a pumping action—these two valves close and prevent blood from returning to the atriums. Remember, the flow of blood only moves in one direction.

Interesting fact! When the valves malfunction and the blood does flow back, this is called *valvular insufficiency*. Now you're one step closer to mesmerizing your in-laws during the next Christmas dinner.

What happens when the ventricles finish contracting and the blood is pumped away to the body and lungs? You're absolutely right! They relax, allow fresh blood to flow in, and get ready for the next pumping action. When this happens, we can't allow all that pressurized blood to return to the ventricle, can we?

This is where the next two valves come in. These are called *semilunar valves,* as they have the distinctive shape of a half-moon. These bad boys close during the relaxation of the ventricles, preventing all that highly pressurized blood from flowing back because, as you remember, the pumping action has to go only in one direction.

If you're really curious, the right semilunar valve is called the *pulmonary valve*. The left one is called the *aortic valve*.

Every single muscle in our body needs blood to function properly. Our heart—the big boss that drives this hydraulic system, is no exception. Naturally, the heart gets the VIP treatment when it comes to a fresh supply of blood. Right above the aortic valve, two dedicated blood vessels are ready to provide the heart with much-needed blood. They are called *coronary arteries*. As you may have guessed, there's a left and a right one. Each one is responsible for servicing its dedicated side of the heart.

Have you ever wondered why bulletproof vests have such a distinctive shape? They are designed to protect our vital organs, mainly our heart and lungs. Nature also did its best to protect these vital organs. Just like our brain is surrounded by hard bones, our heart and lungs are protected by a bony cage—the ribs. This bony cage is called the *thorax*. In the thorax, our heart is happily nestled neatly in between our lungs. This place is called the *mediastinum*. The heart wouldn't be the heart if it wasn't surrounded by its own separate layer of tissue called the *pericardium.* The pericardium is connected to the cavities of the lungs, our diaphragm, and our esophagus.

If this all sounds complicated, think of all this tissue as an anchor that firmly holds our "blood engine" in its place. Nature thought of everything. Even between our heart and the pericardium, there's a thin layer of liquid that allows the heart to contract and relax even more freely. If this isn't VIP treatment, I don't know what is.

Let's take a moment to absorb all this information:

- There are in fact two heart pumps neatly settled inside one organ.
- The atriums don't handle great blood pressure, while the ventricles do.
- The left atrium and ventricle system provides blood to our entire body.
- The right system provides blood only to our lungs.
- The valves ensure that the blood flow only goes in one direction.
- The heart has its own special housing inside the thorax, called the pericardium.

Now you know the basic building blocks of our heart. You know your atriums, ventricles, valves, and arteries. Well done! Let's continue and take an even closer look at the physiology of the heart. This is something even more fascinating.

PHYSIOLOGY OF THE HEART

If you're wondering what the word *physiology* means, it's simply "the study of how an organ functions." In this section we'll examine a bit closer how exactly our heart works. Not only will it be extremely fascinating, but it will also give you a better understanding of heart diseases and current treatments that exist today. Again, don't feel intimidated by all the medical complexity! We'll take everything one step at a time and do our best to explain every minute detail.

Heartbeat

Diastole

Systole

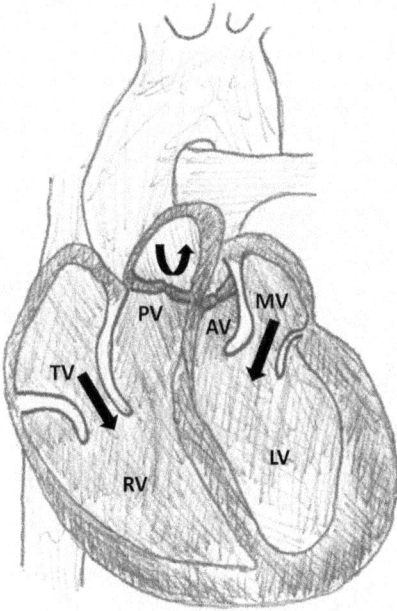
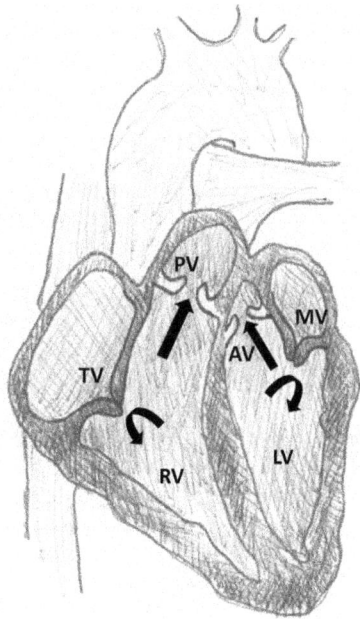

Figure 4.
During diastole, the relaxation of the heart muscle, the heart chambers fill with blood. Blood flows into the left (LV) and right ventricle (RV), the tricuspid (TV) and mitral valve (MV) are open. The semilunar valves are closed.
During systole, the contraction of the heart muscle, the blood is ejected over the aortic (AV) and pulmonary valve (PV) to the systemic and pulmonary circulation. The atrioventricular valves are closed.

As you remember from the previous chapter, when the atriums and ventricles contract, blood gets expelled out of the heart—in the same way a classic bellow mechanism blows our air when you press it together. This muscle contraction is called *systole*. Naturally, every contraction is followed by relaxation. When the muscle relaxes, we call this *diastole*.

During systole (contraction), blood is pressurized and sent to the arteries. On the other hand, during diastole (relaxation), the atriums

Conduction system of the heart

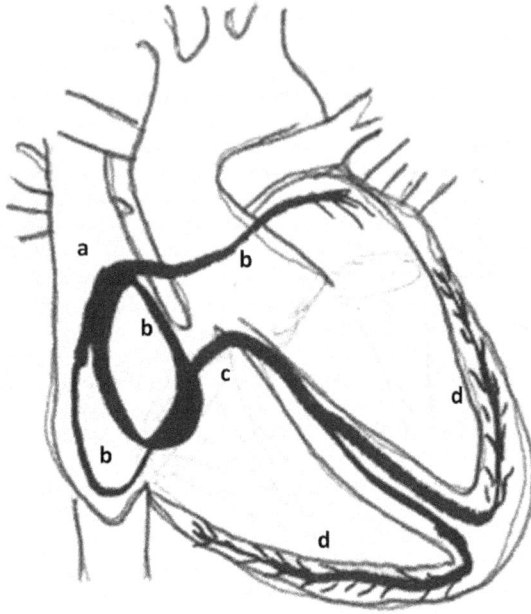

Figure 5.
The impulse to trigger the heartbeat originates in the sinus node (a). It spreads over the atriums through atrial conduction pathways (b) and reaches the atrioventricular node(c). The atrioventricula node brings the signal to the ventricular conduction pathways (d) that trigger the ventricular contraction, called systole.

and ventricles are filled with fresh blood. So, how does the heart know when to contract and when to relax? There are special cells that generate an impulse that drives the process of systole. These cells are notoriously hard workers, and they activate about sixty times per minute on average. They live in a tight cluster at the entrance of the right atrium in what is called the *sinus node*.

When the signal impulse is generated, it gets propagated by special pathways, only to spread further throughout the atriums and ventricles—triggering their contraction and subsequent pumping action. Just like after hard work comes relaxation, so is systole followed up by diastole.

During diastole, our heart muscles are relaxed and welcome the next delivery of fresh blood into the heart. At the end of diastole, the heart is relaxed to the maximum capacity and can hold a respectable 120 ml of blood inside the left ventricle alone. Subsequently, after the heart muscle contracts and sends all this blood on its way throughout our body, about 50 ml of blood remains in the left ventricle. As you can see, the heart works with an efficiency of about 60 percent. In other words, during every systole, 60 percent of the blood volume present in the left ventricle will be ejected to the arteries.

This proportion of ejected blood is called the *ejection fraction*, and it happens to be one of the most important parameters that we can use to examine a properly functioning heart.

During systole, the heart also pressurizes the blood. This blood pressure that our heart generates plays a major role in our cardiovascular system. The pressure ensures that our blood circulates throughout our entire body. Again, let's think about the basic principles of hydrodynamics; when we want to circulate a liquid across a network of pipes and tubes, we need to crank up the pressure to overcome the natural resistance and "friction" along the way. The laws of physics always apply, remember?

The word *pressure* instinctively associates with standard units of measurement such as bar and Pascal of pressure per square inch (PSI). In the medical field we like to pay tribute to the old-school ways. In the past, blood pressure was measured visually with the help of a simple device—a vessel filled with mercury with a small glass tube attached to it. The patient's blood pressure would translate to rising mercury levels inside a glass tube. This rising mercury level was measured in millimeters. Hence, the OG method of measuring blood pressure today remains millimeters of mercury (mmHg).

Our right ventricle only services our lungs and therefore requires a lower pressure to achieve a respectable 5 liters of blood flow every

Old-school blood pressure measurement device

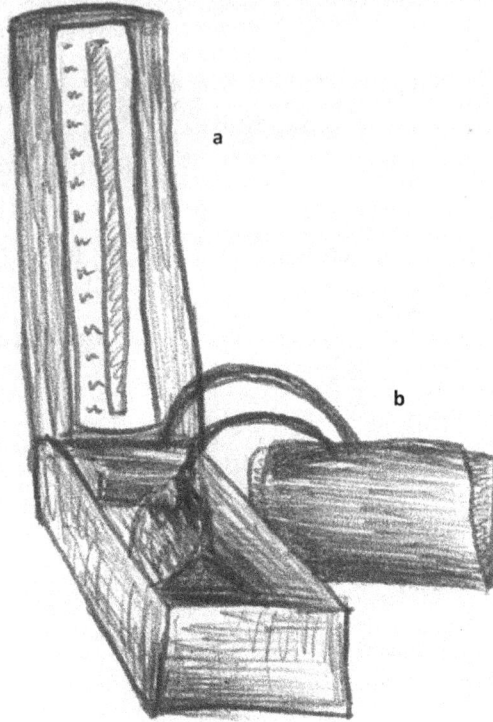

Figure 6.
Blood pressure measurement with a column of mercury (a). The pressure cuff (b) is inflated while wrapped around your upper arm. The corresponding pressure in the cuff is shown by the level of mercury in the column. With a stethoscope the physician will listen to the blood vessels at the level of your elbow. Whilst listening, the pressure in the cuff will be released gently. When he starts to hear the blood pumping the corresponding pressure is the systolic pressure as the sound fades again that is your diastolic blood pressure

minute. The pressure is also lower—about 20 millimeters of mercury (mmHg). The big brother on the left side, that services our entire body, needs to cough up an awesome 120 mmHg of pressure during systole (i.e., the contraction of the left ventricle). Naturally, these measurements will vary, simply because our heart adapts its function to the requirements of the body. How does the heart muscle know exactly how fast and how strong it needs to contract at any given time?

You see, there are several very clever regulatory systems that help guide our heart and help it to work properly. Some of these systems are nestled in the heart itself. Other systems use a complex array of nerves and hormones to send signals remotely. In general, these systems can help increase the flow rate of our blood by regulating just two variables: the speed of our heartbeat and the power of muscle contractions of the heart itself.

The rate of contractions of the heart muscle is regulated by the sinoatrial node. If the cells in this node get stimulated by certain nerves or hormones, they can increase the rate of impulses, hence increasing your heartbeat. Your heart can crank up the speed, but of course it has limits! The maximum frequency of heart muscle contractions can be calculated with a simple formula: 220 minus your age (in years).

An average twenty-year-old person (220 - 20) can reach a respectable 200 heartbeats per minute. An eighty-year-old individual (220 - 80) would have to be satisfied with 140 heartbeats per minute. Of course, a faster heartbeat is possible to achieve. However, this usually requires further examination since this is considered abnormal. If you suddenly feel a compulsory need to stop reading and calculate your own maximum number of heart beats per minute, please feel free to do it! After you have satisfied your curiosity, let's continue.

The opposite can also happen. Some nerves will rock the sinoatrial node to sleep instead of putting it in overdrive. Ever heard of the vagus nerve? When it stimulates the sinoatrial node, it can even decrease the heart rate so much that you will faint. That's why it's called a *vasovagal syncope*.

Other nerves and hormones will unlock the hidden power reserve in your heart muscle fibers, making them work harder to circulate more blood through your body. Let's take a moment to zoom out and look at the amazingly complex biological machine that is our own body. What does it require to function properly? Our blood circulates around our body, delivering oxygen to all the tissues and organs. Aside from that, our blood also collects carbon dioxide and waste material and carries them to the designated organs for proper disposal.

Our body strives for perfect balance, so naturally, our blood keeps the concentration of all those substances in a constant state of equilibrium. Let's imagine that one of your organs suddenly needs more oxygen. This simply means that this very organ needs a bit more blood flow—hence, the heart will have to kick into a higher gear. For example, when you're pumping iron in the gym or doing other sports, doubling or tripling your cardiac output is not uncommon. When you're vegging on your sofa and watching Netflix, this rate decreases to just 5 l/min. In short—a perfect equilibrium!

Let's recap what we know so far:

- Heart contraction is called systole.
- Heart relaxation is called diastole.
- During every systole 60 percent of the volume is pushed out of the ventricle. This is called the ejection fraction.
- In rest, our heart pumps 5 l/min of blood. During exercise this can go up to 20 l/min.
- Pumping more is achieved by faster and stronger contractions of the muscle.

THE HEART MUSCLE

Now that we know a bit more about the physiology of our heart, let's dive a bit deeper into how our heart muscle actually works. This is extremely fascinating! By now you hopefully still remember that our heart is a very special muscle. Muscles are present everywhere in our body. The muscles that you can consciously manipulate are called *skeletal muscles*. As you may have guessed, they are indeed attached to your skeleton. When you pick up a glass of water or turn a page in this book, these muscles are under your command. They work whenever you give them a command to do so.

If you're really curious, on a microscopic level these are called the *striated muscles*. They have a distinctive tubular shape, several nuclei per fiber, and in some parts of our body they can reach a whopping ten

16

centimeters in length. Each muscle fiber is controlled separately by our nerve dendrites that branch out from our nerve cells. There are plenty of them, and they are all interconnected—one muscle needs many different nerve cells to function properly. Why is that?

We may not even think about it, but our skeletal muscles need to work with high precision—with full ability to handle complex tasks. This means that when a muscle contracts, it doesn't always contract completely and at full force. This is made possible by the dendrites that control each fiber individually, creating tiny movements of a large muscle. This is why chefs can skillfully navigate a knife just a few millimeters from their fingers, musicians can blindly position their fingers anywhere on the fretboard of their guitar, and surgeons can perform delicate cuts and stitches without endangering the life of their patients.

Our skeletal muscle cells are tightly bound with special connective tissue that ends in a tendon—securely connected to our bones. This marriage between muscle and bone results in the ability to transfer power and motion to our body.

While our arms, legs, and fingers are under our direct control, there are several other bodily functions we are never aware of. In fact, our body is full of muscles that seem to work on autopilot—without our direct input. These muscles are called the *smooth muscles*. When you send a delicious meal to your stomach, your stomach muscles contract and relax—making quick work of digestion. The same happens inside the intestines when they work hard to move the nutrients down the entire gastrointestinal system. Even the airways to our lungs, as well as tiny muscles that are attached to our blood vessels, are in a constant state of contraction and relaxation. Your body does all this tedious work without bothering your consciousness about it. Can you even begin to imagine what a nightmare it would be if you had to consciously control all these muscles every minute?

Without these so-called smooth muscles, our body would cease to exist. If you really want to know why they are called smooth muscles, it's simply because they lack the distinctive tubular structure that's typical for our skeletal muscles. Smooth muscles are pretty special as well. You see, they have just one cell nucleus that's nestled neatly inside the center of the muscle fiber itself. These muscles are also smaller in comparison to skeletal muscles. Rightfully so, because as you remember, we cannot consciously manipulate them at will. The contraction and relaxation motion of the smooth muscles is made possible with the help of nerves and hormones.

How do the skeletal muscles and smooth muscles compare to our heart? Our heart muscle fibers are quite different from anything else in our body. In medicine we call the heart muscles *cardiomyocytes*. Again, don't let the strange-sounding jargon intimidate you! This is a simple combination of two words—*cardia* (heart) and *myocyte* (muscle cell).

When it comes to their design, cardiomyocytes share the same tubular pattern as our skeletal muscles, but they are much smaller in overall size. What makes our heart muscle so different is the connection between all the separate muscle cells. This connection is mechanically perfect and rock solid.

You see, this allows for easy propagation of mechanical forces, as well as electric impulses. In essence, when just a single muscle cell receives an electrical impulse, this is enough to initiate the contraction of our entire heart! This amazingly efficient electrical conductivity system allows every impulse to propagate through the heart muscle in a neatly coordinated way. So, in contrast to a skeletal muscle, where each fiber is controlled separately and thus can contract independently, the heart muscle works as a whole. One electrical signal and the entire heart will contract! How does this look in practice?

We already know that when a muscle contracts, it becomes shorter. When it relaxes, it should theoretically return to its original length, right? Unfortunately, it is a bit more complicated. When our muscles relax, they are in fact being "pulled" back to the original state of relaxation. Inside the skeletal muscles, this happens by the antagonist. This is simply a muscle that pulls in a different direction. This is achieved by the muscles that are connected to our joints.

For example, when you stretch out your arm, your triceps muscle is pulling, while your biceps is relaxed. In fact, your triceps ensures that your biceps is "pulled" into a state of total relaxation. When you bend your arm, the exact opposite effect takes place. Now the biceps muscle is "pulling," while your triceps muscle is relaxed. Pretty logical, right?

Let's look at our heart for a second. There is not a single antagonist muscle to be found! The heart muscle is one single unit. So how can it reach the Valhalla of total relaxation? This is where the fibrous skeleton of the heart enters the scene. Again, let's not get lost in the medical jargon. Of course, there's no skeleton inside our heart. The secret is in the design of our heart valves.

You see, our four heart valves are suspended in a solid ring of connective tissue. Those four rings are nestled very close together and form a solid base—anchoring the muscular wall of the atriums and ventricles firmly in place. So there is a solid base to contract against but still no antagonist. Luckily our heart has another amazing design feature. Between the muscular cells of our heart there's a special elastic tissue. It acts like a natural spring mechanism. After every heartbeat, this elastic tissue ensures that the muscular fibers "bounce back" into their original position. The result of this mechanical perfection is that our cardiomyocytes are neatly "pulled" back into their original state of total relaxation.

While your skeletal muscles have ample time to be pulled back into their original state of relaxation, the heart muscle cannot afford such a luxury. Luckily, thanks to the amazing design of the valve rings and the elastic tissue, our cardiomyocytes can now relax immediately, allowing the atriums and ventricles to be filled back up with the well-needed blood, ready to be pumped to wherever it's needed in our body. Fun fact: this filling process happens passively, because as you remember, the heart is relaxed.

Let's look at the fibrous skeleton a bit closer. It has another trick up its sleeve. It forms an electrical insulation between atriums and ventricles. This creates a slight delay between the atrial and ventricular contraction. Why is this needed?

Cardiac cycle

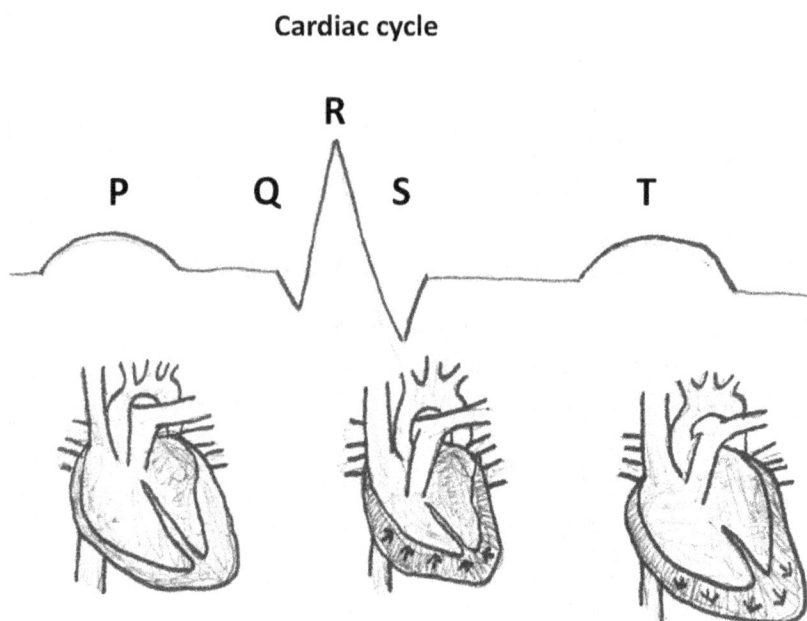

Figure 7.
ECG of a heart beat (top) with corresponding contraction states of the heart (bottom). The P wave corresponds to the contraction of the atriums. The QRS wave corresponds to the ventricular contraction (systole). The delay between P and QRS wave is caused by the atrioventricular node and ventricular conduction pathways, allowing for optimal ventricular filling. The T wave indicates the relaxation of the ventricles (diastole), this completes the cardiac cycle. After a short interval the cardiac cycle will repeat.

Simply put, to ensure the optimal fill rate of our ventricles—the hard workers of our heart. The entire process is quite straightforward. First, the ventricles relax and fill passively with blood from the atriums. Second, the atriums contract and squeeze out the last blood to the ventricles to fill them up to the maximum capacity. Only then can the ventricle contract and send the blood away to our body. We cannot help but marvel at the efficiency of our heart. But wait, there's more!

The cardiomyocytes of our ventricles are very well organized. They form a helical shape starting from the tip of our heart, down to the fibrous skeleton at the very bottom. When our heart muscle contracts, the ventricles not only pump the blood away but are also "wrung out" in the same way you would wring out a wet T-shirt after a well-needed wash. Now you know just how efficient our heart really is. Let's take a moment to let the new knowledge gestate before we continue.

BLOOD CIRCULATION

As you remember from the previous sections, our blood is a truly magnificent liquid of life that performs different vital functions in our body. It's well worth expanding on this topic a bit deeper.

Just like the water in your house, blood also flows through pipes. We call them *blood vessels*. There are two types of blood vessels. Those taking blood to the heart are called *veins* (low-pressure pipes), and those taking it away from the heart are the *arteries* (high-pressure pipes).

Let's follow our blood as it returns from our organs to our heart. We start with the blood that likes to hang out in our venous system. Just like all roads lead to Rome, so does the venous system—a network of veins that eventually comes back to our heart. Look at the back of your hands. Do you see all the small veins?

All of these veins will eventually come together at the entrance of your right atrium and find their way to the right ventricle. From there the blood will move on to your lungs to dispatch all the nasty carbon dioxide and collect fresh oxygen. Now that the blood is nice and oxygenated, it will flow via the lung veins straight into the left atrium on its way to the big boss of the heart, the left ventricle. When the left ventricle contracts, it sends this blood to all the organs and tissues that are by now gasping for fresh oxygen.

After the blood visits all the tissues and organs, it's time to head back into the veins that lead back into the right atrium and ventricle and subsequently to the lungs. As you may have guessed, this makes a perfect closed loop.

Pulmonary and systemic circulation

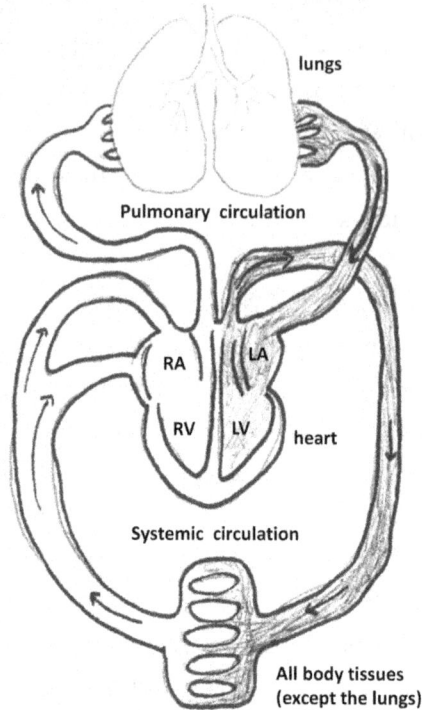

Figure 8.

The pulmonary circulation starts at the right ventricle (RV) and brings the deoxygenated blood (white) to the lungs. After passing through the lungs, the oxygenated blood (dark) flows to the left atrium (LA).

The systemic circulation starts at the left venticle (LV) and brings the oxygenated blood (dark) to all the organs and tissues of our body by means of our arteries. The deoxygenated blood (white) is brought back to the right atrium (RA) by the veins.

The blood flow that starts from the right ventricle and ends at the left atrium is called the *lesser* or *pulmonary circulation*. As you remember, this highway takes the blood only to the lungs (*pulmo*= "lung"), eventually finishing at the left side of our heart.

The blood that exits the left ventricle, passes our entire body, and eventually ends up back in the right atrium is called the *greater* or *systemic circulation*. If we want to imagine just how great it is, this circulatory system needs to pass through many different arteries only to visit all our vital tissues and organs. In essence, both the pulmonary and systemic circulation are connected in series. First the blood needs to pass the pulmonary circulation, and then it's ready for the systemic circulation.

When we mention artificial heart pumps, they are almost always connected to our systemic circulation. We'll explain why and how very soon, I promise. First, it's very interesting to examine a few important blood vessels that happen to be vital when we are working with these heart pumps. Ready?

Even if you are a newbie in the medical field, you probably know the aorta. This is the biggest vessel in our body. With a whopping diameter of 2.5 cm (almost a full inch), the aorta is the first artery that welcomes pressurized blood from the left ventricle. As you may remember, the semilunar valve prevents blood from returning to the left ventricle during diastole (when the heart relaxes). In essence, it ensures that the blood only flows in one direction—from the ventricle to the artery and never in reverse. Can you guess what this valve is called? Of course, it's the aortic valve! Let's follow it and see where we end up.

About 15 cm down into the aorta, we can see a few very important arteries branching out. They welcome blood flow to both of our arms and to our head. The arteries designated for our arms are located under our clavicles. They pass our armpits and arrive at their destination in the arms. If you're curious, the artery that's located right under your armpit is called the *axillary artery* (*axilla* = "armpit").

Now that we have supplied our arms and head with blood, what happens to the aorta? It takes a sharp turn south and moves down toward our lower body. Our spine is the perfect armor for such an important "blood highway," so naturally, the aorta will follow alongside our spine toward our abdomen. Now that our vital organs are supplied with much-needed oxygenated blood, we can split up the blood flow to address the needs of our legs. These important arteries are located in our groin area, and they are called *femoral arteries*.

The aorta, axillary arteries, and femoral arteries are quite important to remember. Why? First, they are located in perfectly strategic

Main arteries of the systemic circulation

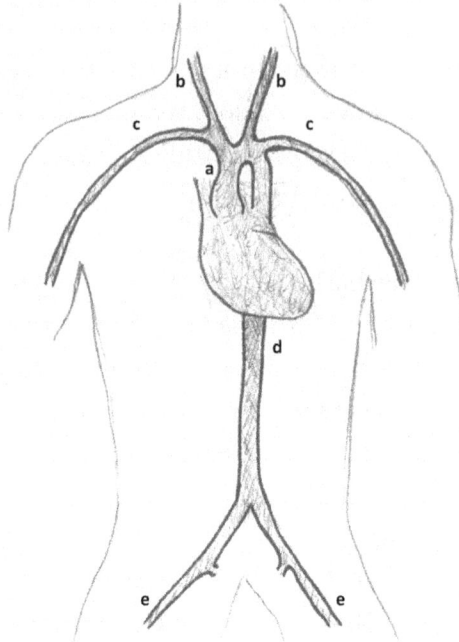

Figure 9.
The ascending aorta (a) leaves the heart and ascends to the neck region. Branches towards the head, the carotid arteries (b) and arms, the axillary arteries (c) take off. Now the aorta takes a turn to descend (d) again towards the abdomen. At the level of your umbilicus the aorta branches and the femoral arteries (e) will supply blood to the legs.

areas. This allows surgeons fast access—which can mean the difference between life and death. Of course, the large size of these arteries plays a major factor as well. The aorta is the biggest artery in our body, yet the other two can be equally proud of their quite respectable size—almost 1 cm in diameter. Can we by any chance use these three blood superhighways for connecting artificial pumps? Absolutely!

Let's quickly recap!

- Veins bring blood to the heart—the blood pressure is low.
- Arteries bring blood to the tissues and organs; they run away

from the heart and have high blood pressure.

- The greater circulation, also called *systemic circulation,* brings blood to all the organs and tissues.
- The lesser circulation, also called *pulmonary circulation,* services only the lungs.
- The aorta, axillary arteries, and femoral arteries are the ones that surgeons prefer to use for connecting an artificial pump to your systemic circulation.

A WORD ABOUT OUR BLOOD

Our heart—as well as artificial heart pumps—circulate blood throughout our body every minute of every day. Let's take a moment to examine this liquid of life. After this chapter you'll gain a better understanding of the interaction between our blood and artificial heart pumps. Naturally, you'll also understand a few potential side effects. Well-informed is well-armed! One thing I can promise you is that after this chapter, you will never be scared of 1980s-style horror films ever again.

You may see blood as a liquid. However, it's also an entire organ with its own cells and functions. A respectable 45 percent of blood is composed of cells. The other 55 percent is a liquid solution of many interesting substances, called *plasma*. This concoction of cells, proteins, and plasma makes blood rather viscous or thick, almost like a syrup. This thickness is called *viscosity*, which can be measured.

When we happen to have plenty of red blood cells drifting around our blood vessels, our blood is considered more viscous. The opposite is also true; fewer red blood cells mean more liquid blood. Let's grab a microscope and look at our blood a bit closer. We'll quickly discover that there are three main types of blood cells.

We have already met the red blood cells. They look like small, flat discs without a nucleus. These tiny hard workers love to transport oxygen as well as carbon dioxide. Life without oxygen is impossible; therefore, it's quite self-explanatory that we have many red blood cells in our body. At any given moment there can be as many as five billion of these tiny workers living inside just 1 milliliter of blood.

If you're curious, the protein called *hemoglobin* is the magic ingredient that allows our red blood cells to transport oxygen. This amazing hemoglobin also contains iron—giving our blood a distinctive red color. This is definitely something to remember when you watch your next horror film.

The second group of cells we can spot under the microscope are called *blood platelets*. For the sake of accuracy, these are not cells, but rather small pieces that originate from bigger cells in our bone marrow. These bigger cells shedding small platelets are so big, scientists named them *megakaryocytes*. Pretty cool to be called mega, no? Whenever you cut your finger, be sure to thank these megakaryocytes (and, of course, other proteins) for allowing your blood to clot—closing up your nasty cut as if by the stroke of a magic wand. If you want to know just how important platelets are, consider this: when we have too few of them floating around in our blood, we can start seeing nasty spontaneous hemorrhages.

The third group is our white blood cells. If you remember high school biology, these cells are the soldiers that guard us from infections. Aside from these three types of cells, what else can we find in our blood?

Let's not forget that our blood contains a plethora of interesting proteins and other substances that all serve their specific purposes. Nature thought of everything! Although we can go a lot deeper into all blood functions, it's important to focus on what's most relevant to us and the topic of this book.

As you remember, our blood can clot in order to seal wounds. This life-saving gift is made possible with the help of special proteins. One of these amazing proteins is called the *von Willebrand factor*. We will expand on this later on.

As the icing on the cake, let's not forget the final important functions of our blood—the ability to transport nutrients and regulate hormones and ions. There are also special proteins that make all of this possible. Our blood is a very complex organ, and we cannot help but marvel at its perfection.

CHAPTER 2

DISEASES OF OUR HEART

MANY PEOPLE MISTAKENLY BELIEVE THAT ALL HEART issues originate from our own—often unhealthy—lifestyle. Nothing can be further from the truth! Many heart conditions are related to an unhealthy lifestyle, but some have nothing to do with your diet or physical fitness. In fact, there are a whole plethora of different heart diseases and abnormalities. Sadly these issues are quite frequent, and this is exactly why we should discuss them. Here we are exploring issues with the heart muscle, the valves, and even the conductive systems that convey electrical impulses.

In some instances, an artificial heart pump can be a literal lifesaver. In others, it is completely unnecessary. As a rule of thumb, when your heart ceases to pump enough blood to the body, only then can we start considering an artificial heart pump as a viable option.

As we dive deeper into this chapter, we will examine the most frequently occurring syndromes and diseases that can eventually lead toward disruptions in the normal pumping action of our heart. Although there are many ways to classify heart diseases, for the sake of simplicity, let's classify them into just two groups: congenital and acquired.

As you may imagine, the word *congenital* simply means the heart is already different from the moment you arrive in this world. When it comes to acquired diseases, they love to rear their ugly head during the later stage of our (sometimes unhealthy and sedentary) life. When you're treating your body like a dumpster, expect to see these horsemen of your very own personal health apocalypse show up on your doorstep, guns blazing. You have been warned!

CONGENITAL HEART DEFECTS

As you may have guessed, there are many congenital heart defects out there, and they range in severity. There are small and harmless situations, where your heart functions may not be affected at all. For example, some patients have a small hole in the interventricular septum—the wall that divides our ventricles. Today two to six people out of one thousand share this condition, and usually this is solved with a simple operation. In other cases, this operation is not necessary at all, and the patient can look forward to a long, happy, and fulfilling life.

On the other hand, there are some instances where the congenital heart defect is quite serious indeed. Some young patients will require several operations to rectify these heart conditions. Even after the surgeons do everything in their power to help a child with a congenital heart defect, there's still a very real, lingering probability that at some point, the heart will fail to pump blood as normal. Usually this happens when the child has already matured into a fully formed adult man or woman.

In the medical field, we have learned a great deal over the past decades. The art of congenital heart surgery has been practiced since the 1950s and 1960s—leading toward the development of life-saving surgeries for children and adults all over the world. In some ways, these people are insanely lucky to be alive. We even coined a new term for them—GUCH (*grown-up congenital heart*). Let's take a look at a classic example.

Sometimes a baby is born with two major arteries (the aorta and the pulmonary artery) that are completely switched and subsequently connected to the wrong ventricles. Hopefully you still remember that

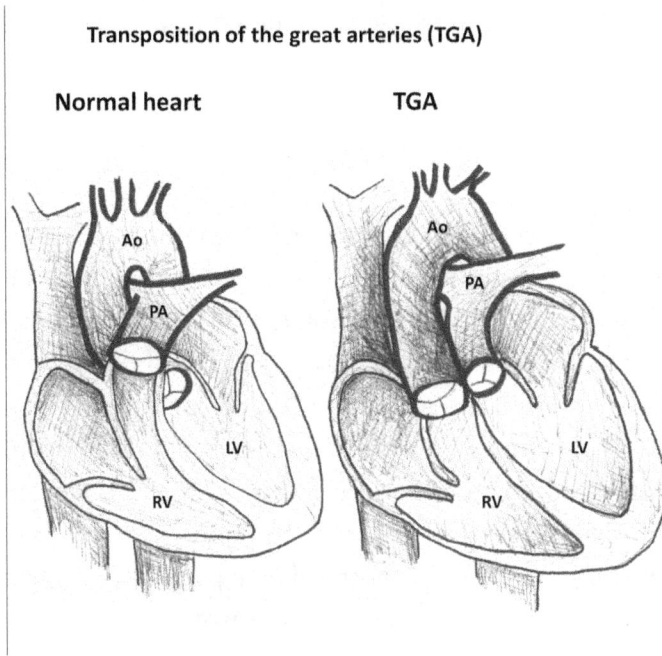

Transposition of the great arteries (TGA)

Normal heart   **TGA**

Figure 10.
In a Transposition of the great arteries (TGA), the pulmonary artery (PA) originates from the left ventricle (LV) instead of the right ventricle (RV). The aorta (Ao), on the other hand, originates from the right ventricle (RV). This configuration makes the right ventricle the pump for the systemic circulation, while the left ventricle will service the pulmonary circulation.

the aorta is normally connected to the "big boss" left ventricle, while the pulmonary artery is connected to the right one. In this case, both arteries are switched—transposed.

As you may remember from the past chapters, our blood flow is always moving in series like this:

Left atrium > Left ventricle > **Body** > Right atrium > Right ventricle > **Lungs** > Left atrium again . . .

The cycle is complete when the blood visits all four parts of our heart, the lungs, and the body—delivering all that heavily oxygenated blood to every nook and cranny of our body. Oxygen is life, and we need plenty of it to be happy and healthy.

When we are dealing with a transposition of the great arteries (TGA), we're literally looking at two separate blood flows that are working in parallel:

Blood flow nr.1

Right ventricle > **Body** > Right atrium > Right ventricle again

Blood flow nr. 2

Left ventricle > **Lungs** > Left atrium > Left ventricle again

If you want a simple and blunt summary, this congenital heart defect is a death sentence! First, there is absolutely no possibility of providing oxygen to the systemic circulation as blood from the lungs enters the pulmonary circulation again. Indeed, blood coming from the lungs goes to the left atrium and ventricle and through the misconnected pulmonary artery to the lungs again! Oxygen is life, and every single organ in our body needs it—without exception!

The cherry on top is that our left and right parts of the heart, built to handle different flow and pressure, are now working in the completely wrong way. The big boss left ventricle is servicing the pulmonary circulation, while the weaker and more fragile right ventricle must work overtime to provide an ample supply of blood to the entire body via systemic circulation. Without any exaggeration, a tiny patient with this condition would be having a very, *very* bad time, and we have to help them immediately.

Today this heart defect is corrected by switching the arteries to their designated position. The aorta is connected to the left ventricle and the pulmonary artery to the right ventricle. In the past, this was done a bit differently—we diverted the blood flow from the right atrium to the left ventricle. On the other side, the blood flow from the left atrium was diverted to the right ventricle. Once both heart pumps are finally connected in series, oxygenated blood starts cruising throughout the body. But before you exhale a sigh of relief, let's not forget that the roles of the ventricles are still switched!

The big boss left ventricle is servicing the lungs, while the small brother, the right ventricle, is huffing and puffing just to pump the blood across the entire body. Remember, our ventricles are built for the right job, and unfortunately, in this scenario, they are performing quite opposite functions. We are dealing with completely different blood pressure and flow here. As much as we would like it, we can't cheat physics.

Over time, our heart will adapt to this new, somewhat strange reality. The right ventricle will become a more powerful, hairy-chested athlete. A patient can happily live well into their thirties and forties with this condition. In some cases, even fifty-year-old patients can step into the spotlight to tell their story. Yet, like all good stories come to an end, so will the function of the right ventricle. It's just not cut out for such a serious task, so the heart will start to fail, and our patient will need surgical help once again. The good news is that the death sentence that nature dealt to our patients can now be corrected—reason enough to pop the cork of a champagne bottle!

Now that we know a little more about congenital transposition, let's examine another congenital heart defect. Sometimes a patient can be born with just one ventricle, which would require a series of surgeries to correct. We call these surgeries the *Fontan procedure*. As you may imagine, the single lonely ventricle has to push itself over the limit to provide blood to both lungs and the body. Over time, this will unfortunately lead to heart failure, though sometimes patients live past twenty or thirty years before the onset of heart failure comes knocking on the front door.

Today, many people happily live with an artificial heart pump, with the two above-mentioned examples of serious heart defects making up a very small minority of these patients. I've had the honor of working on many of these special cases, and every single one is truly unique. Let's take a sidestep and meet one of the patients, shall we?

Meet Lucas! If you pass him on the street, you'll see an average thirty-two-year-old man. If you stopped to shake his hand, it would never even cross your mind that Lucas was born with a congenital transposition of the great arteries.

Naturally, this means he had to undergo a serious surgical procedure as a baby. Surgeons worked tirelessly to bypass his blood flow from the left atrium to the right ventricle. At the same time, the blood flow from the right atrium was bypassed to his left ventricle. The result? Lucas has been given another chance at life! For now, at least . . .

As the years went by, the baby Lucas became a playful toddler and eventually a strapping young lad. He was simply crushing it! His school days were handled with a healthy dose of youthful defiance, while his free time was filled with mischief and partying. Not many people know this, but Belgium is quite famous for its amazing beer. The golden hoppy nectar is more than just a proud aspect of our heritage—it almost borders on religion. Being a proud Belgian, Lucas definitely kept up with friends at the parties. In the meantime, his heart worked tirelessly to keep up with his shenanigans . . .

As time licked his wounds and taught him some well-needed wisdom, Lucas decided to focus on his education. He buried his nose in books and courses, and even found the time to fall in love with a girl that eventually became his wife. After graduation, Lucas eagerly started his professional career, and shortly after, the happy couple got married. It doesn't take long until the newlyweds welcome a third member of their small family—a healthy baby girl.

At the age of twenty-seven, our hero seemed to be leading a perfectly normal life. However, we know Lucas was a bit different from most of his friends, so there were some things he had to keep in mind. It was perfectly fine for him to go out with friends for some beers, but a wild, adrenaline-filled weekend was not something his heart could handle. Lucas was a wonderful dad and could change diapers like a boss, but when it came to goofing around while pushing his daughter in a stroller, this duty was handled by Mom. Riding a bike was fine, as long as it had an electric motor that could help.

These inconveniences certainly didn't prevent Lucas from having a rich, happy, and fulfilling life. For twenty-seven years straight, his heart did a great job keeping him alive. However, the right ventricle was fighting a constantly losing battle—as you remember it was not designed for the kinds of pressure and blood flow it was currently dealing with. Lucas, of course, noticed this alarming trend as well, and it was impossible for him to know how much time he would be blessed with before his next inevitable operation. We'll return to Lucas's story later.

As you can see, though congenital heart defects used to mean a literal death sentence by nature, today, people with these conditions often receive a second chance at having a truly fulfilling life. Luckily, these cases are quite rare. In most cases of failing hearts, we are dealing with a perfectly normal heart that has been stricken with illness or another condition that severely damaged all the normal heart functions. Let's learn about these acquired heart conditions.

ACQUIRED HEART CONDITIONS

As much as we wish for it, we're not immortal, and every one of us can be stricken with illness at any moment. Sometimes it's the heart muscle itself that starts to act up. This naturally leads toward a decreased ability to pump blood across our entire body. In other cases, our heart valves or even the electric conduction system can be the source of our misery. When these systems are out of balance, we can see overstimulation and overload of our heart muscle. Our body has an amazing ability to compensate for some loss of an organs function, but there are limits to this process. In summary, these complex and quite destructive processes usually take many years to metastasize inside our body. With the help of well-chosen treatment, life can now be prolonged for a lot longer than ever before. Let's go ahead and meet some of the usual suspects.

Ischemic cardiomyopathies—lack of blood supply to the heart muscle
It is one of the most frequent heart conditions out there. It's the culprit disease in more than half of our patients with a heart pump. But I hear you thinking, what the hell does *ischemic cardiomyopathy* mean?

Don't worry, again we won't allow ourselves to be intimidated by the medical jargon. Instead, let's take a moment to understand this condition. There are many cases when our coronary arteries become constricted. This is called *ischemic heart disease*. Now, what is *ischemia*? Simply put, it refers to oxygen shortage in our organs. In our case, we're talking about Monsieur Heart Muscle himself.

When we're referring to conditions whereby our heart muscle is experiencing issues (any type of issues), we call this *cardiomyopathy*. When we're talking about ischemic cardiomyopathy, we of course refer to the issues with the heart muscle caused by oxygen shortage. That's it! Now we have dispatched all the complexity, the natural question worth asking is, how can our coronary arteries become constricted in the first place? In order to answer this question, we will have to have a critical look at our own lifestyle. Ready?

Enter *atherosclerosis*. Fat and cholesterol love to accumulate inside our arteries, causing all kinds of devastation inside our heart and cardiovascular system. Certainly, when you love to smoke cigarettes in between your fat filled meals! At some point these nasty deposits become so large that they can impede blood flow to our heart muscle itself, leading to many nasty issues as a result. To put it bluntly, when your coronary arteries are clogged up by the efforts of your own reck-lessness, your heart won't be able to function properly! When (and how) does this phenomenon usually occur?

It's hard to say, because every case is truly unique. What we do know for sure is that the process of clogging your arteries takes a long time to become noticeable. Usually, when your heart is pumping at a jolly sixty beats per minute, there will still be some oxygenated blood that reaches your heart. However, when you need to grind through serious physical activities—triggering your heart to beat faster and harder—this is where you run into trouble. When your heart beats faster and produces a much higher pumping force, this small amount of blood just won't be enough to feed the machine with oxygen.

The problems will start slowly. Your body will do its best to remind you of your poor lifestyle choices with the help of a heavy, tight, and painful squeezing feeling inside your chest. Doctors call it *angina pectoris*. When the physical stress is reduced and the heart's pumping action can decrease to a lower pace, this alarming feeling in your chest will subside. Our body is amazing at letting us know that something is terribly wrong. It's definitely a good idea not to ignore these serious warnings, but rather to schedule an appointment to have your cardiovascular plumbing checked out. This way you'll have a better understanding of where those nasty constrictions of your arteries are hiding out, growing bigger, and preparing to bite you again when you least expect it.

Depending on the severity of your case and the extend of the diseased coronary arteries, the treatment will usually consist of stents or bypass surgery. Remember, oxygen is life! Our heart muscle needs oxygenated blood to keep us going. What would happen if the constriction in your arteries was so bad that almost no oxygenated blood arrived at your heart muscle? You should definitely sit down to hear this!

Your heart muscle will slowly start to die. Your body will send out alarm signals, and this horrible feeling in your chest will linger even during the moments when your heart is beating slowly. The throbbing pain will wash over many other areas of your body (as the chest pain persists), and you will start to sweat and gasp for breath. You may have already heard about this condition. It's called a *myocardial infarction*. This happened to Michael on the golf course, and believe me when I say it truly feels like the end.

Consider this: even a few minutes into a myocardial infarction, your heart muscle cells will start racking up permanent damage as they become starved of the much-needed oxygen. The more time without oxygen, the greater the damage. Again, you have been warned!

Every case of ischemic cardiomyopathy is unique. Depending on the location of your constricted artery (or arteries), parts of the heart muscle can potentially be lost forever during a myocardial infarction. In some cases, a patient can cheat death with just a bit of heart muscle damage. In other cases, the damage may be greater and much worse. One thing is certain—your heart muscle has just been dragged through pure horror and racked up irreversible tissue damage. Even if your brain can rationalize its way out of your poor life choices, your heart won't forgive you any time soon. Instead, the heart will start to remodel itself to compensate for the new grim reality of living with permanently damaged tissue. What does it look like in practice?

Over the following months and years, there will be some drastically needed changes in your heart. For instance, the remaining heart muscle will need to work overtime just to perform the same duties. The volume of your atriums and ventricles will increase. The muscular walls of your heart will become thicker and stronger. This is called *remodeling,* and this process is necessary to keep you alive. Now, before you get excited and start washing down glazed donuts with a large glass of soda while exhaling a toxic cloud of cigarette smoke, consider the following:

If a healthy heart is a cheetah, capable of running at superhuman speeds, your post-myocardial infarction heart will resemble a lion—strong but sluggish. Even if a small area of your heart muscle becomes stiffer and less nimble, it can lead to an overall worse performance of your entire heart muscle. What's the good news in all of this? With the right treatment and lifestyle, your heart will be thanking you for many decades to come. Someday, it may even forgive you!

This reminds me of one of my patients.

Jan is an active forty-five-year-old man. At the age of eighteen, he started his career in construction. He was a good kid—working hard, yet also finding time to goof around with colleagues during breaks. The fast-paced Belgian lifestyle can take its toll on a man's health. After all, our national dishes are high in calories, fat, and carbohydrates. Our hero was still young, however, and he felt unstoppable—ready to wrestle a bull if he needed to.

He's happily climbed walls and scaled ladders with a lit cigarette dangling from his mouth. During lunch, he eagerly sent a lethal concoction of carbohydrate-rich sandwiches down his esophagus. And at least twice per week, it was time for traditional culinary perversion—real

Belgian fries. If you don't know it yet, the fries that you love so much were invented in Belgium, and to this day, the Belgians make the best fries in the world. The secret is cooking them twice in real beef tallow at varying temperatures. But that's stuff for a completely different book. Let's get back to Jan's story.

Jan's life philosophy was simple—when you work hard, you need plenty of energy! Years flew by, and Jan was happily working as usual. As he passed his fortieth birthday, he began to notice a few subtle changes. When he built a new scaffolding, he noticed that work just "didn't go as jollily as it used to." Sometimes he even needed to stop to take a short break—to catch a breath and let that gnarly tight feeling in his chest subside. Jan brushed it off as "just a part of getting older." Sound familiar?

All would have been well under the sun if not for one strange phenomenon: Jan noticed that his colleagues (who happened to be the same age) didn't share these episodes of fatigue and tightness in the chest. Enough was enough! Playtime was over, and Jan finally decided to take things seriously. On January 2 he was going on a diet—hellbent on losing a hefty thirty kilograms (sixty-six pounds) of excess weight. Just three months and four kilograms of weight loss later, he accepted a crushing defeat. After all, eating bland, tasteless slop was just not worth it—especially when he was not feeling immediate improvement of his health. Screw this!

To add insult to injury, Jan's colleagues didn't make life any easier for him. You see, it's an unspoken international tradition among construction workers to properly tease the hell out of your colleague's "healthy lifestyle." It works even better when you do it while joyfully munching a tasty sandwich during a lunch break. And so, unable to handle the relentless peer pressure, Jan surrendered and returned to his casual dumpster diet. What about the fatigue, shortness of breath, and annoying sensation in his chest? After all, every time he was performing demanding physical labor, these symptoms were never far behind. He simply learned to live with them. As time passed, Jan's colleagues also learned to accept that sometimes Jan just needed to take it easy! That was all it was and there was no reason to panic.

Sometime later Jan was back to his jolly old (overweight) self, happily strolling around with a dangling cigarette and laughing at his colleagues' jokes. However, today, something just feels a bit odd. Jan and his crew are installing an extremely heavy window frame. He's pushing and pulling with all his might, but the damn frame simply refuses to snap into place. Time is running out—the team is hopelessly behind schedule. To make matters worse, Jan's team lead is absent, so this job falls solely and relentlessly on Jan's shoulders. Simply put, he's now in charge of this "bitch of a job."

Hours into this hellish day, Jan's colleagues are completely unaware of his alarmingly dreadful condition. Unbeknownst to everyone, he's been ignoring a serious, tight, oppressive feeling in his chest for almost two hours straight. Stopping to catch his breath right now is a luxury he simply can't afford. Just two more hours, and he's free to head home and take a well-needed rest.

Out of nowhere, the feeling in the chest suddenly morphs into hellish pain. Hot spikes pierce his chest with jolts of electricity. Jan stops in his tracks and sits down. The colleagues notice Jan's blank, emotionless stare as he's gasping for air while the sweat is cascading from his body. Jan's colleagues act quickly, and in mere minutes they deliver him to the emergency room of a nearby hospital. After the painkillers kick in and the much-needed oxygen mask helps his body to stabilize, the doctors decide to run further tests. For Jan, the diagnosis of myocardial infarction echoes like thunder on a sunny day.

Without losing any time, Jan is transferred to another department, where heart specialists begin their meticulous work. Through a small incision in the groin area (*femoral artery*—if you remember correctly), they insert a small flexible tube that leads directly toward Jan's coronary arteries. The worst fear of the doctors is confirmed—one of Jan's coronary arteries is completely blocked. There is no blood flow at all, and a part of his heart muscle has taken some serious punches. The doctors use a stent to open the artery, allowing blood to flow to resume once again.

The next day Jan wakes up, looking and feeling a lot better, gingerly expecting any snippet of good news. The doctors show Jan the blood results and don't hold back as they lay out the severity of his condition:

1. His coronary arteries are constricted, and blood flow is simply abysmal.
2. His heart function has already decreased due to this lack of blood flow.
3. The kidneys are already starting to suffer irreversible damage as well.

This is not a wake-up call. This is the wake-up call!

As of now, it's not a matter of changing his life just to regain the normal strength and stamina needed for work. Unfortunately, it's now a matter of literally keeping his one foot out of the grave. Jan needs to combine a healthy lifestyle with necessary medication—doctor's orders! As the doctors leave his hospital room, the new reality is slowly and painfully seeping in. Today Jan can finally reflect on decades of poor choices staring him right in the face.

He shouldn't have brushed off the obvious symptoms, and he definitely should have listened to his body–the infinitely perfect biological machine that became infuriated by the guy in the driver's seat making one bad decision after the other. As we move further, we'll check back on Jan and see how he's holding up. Now it's time to explore other heart conditions that are well worth knowing about, as maybe someday this knowledge will help you save someone's life.

Valvular cardiomyopathies—Heart Valve Diseases

As you remember, our heart valves ensure that our blood only flows in one direction. When our heart valves malfunction and don't close properly, blood starts flowing back with every heartbeat. Even if the heart muscle itself works flawlessly, eventually your atriums and ventricles will dilate in order to compensate for this phenomenon. Fast-forward a few years, and this will unfortunately cause your heart muscle to fail completely. On the other hand, a valve not opening well can also put a lot of strain on your heart muscle and also lead to a failing heart. The aortic valve especially is at risk of becoming stenotic over time.

We call these conditions *valvular cardiomyopathy*. Although it is quite rare for valve pathology to cascade into overt heart failure, the danger cannot be understated. You see, it takes quite a long time before you notice any issues, as your heart is overcompensating just to keep the blood flow normal. As a patient, you won't feel a thing. By the time you do feel it, the tissue damage might be irreversible.

Heart Failure Due to Arrhythmia—Irregular Heartbeat
A healthy heart that has been beating too fast and working too hard for many years will eventually start to wear out. Most likely culprit here is the so called atrial fibrillation. A condition quite common in the elderly population. Just like with the above-mentioned valvular cardiomy-opathy, arrhythmia is a rather rare cause for irreversible heart failure. Contrary to valvular cardiomyopathy, however, a patient can definitely feel their heart working overtime. Today such an arrhythmia can be treated before it leads to catastrophic heart failure, so it's a good idea to visit a specialist if you feel that something is off. It may save your life!

Nonischemic cardiomyopathies—Heart Failure That Is Unrelated to Oxygen Deprivation
If you remember, ischemic heart failure—when our heart muscle is starved of rich, oxygenated blood—is the primary cause of heart failure by the numbers. However, many patients with ischemic cardiomyop-athy have only a slight degree of heart failure, and there are, in fact, a plethora of illnesses and conditions that can lead toward much more severe heart failure, called *nonischemic cardiomyopathies*. Fortunately, these conditions are rare and are called *nonischemic* just to distinguish them from the large group of ischemic cardiomyopathy without having to invent a name for every disease.

One such example of nonischemic cardiomyopathy is when your heart muscle runs into serious inflammation. A viral infection can simply strike us out of nowhere and cause this condition. This is the famous *myocarditis* that doctors refer to. It's no joke, and in some cases it can cause serious heart damage. Luckily there is light at the end of the tunnel! In many cases this inflammation can subside, and your heart can recover its normal function. Although complete recoveries happen in the majority of cases that we have seen over the years, there can always be tragic exceptions. If by now you may think you have a shot at cheating death and you feel like raising a toast to this occasion, you may want to read on . . .

You don't need to be a doctor to know that toxins wreak havoc on your heart—eventually bringing you a step closer to heart failure. When you're good friends with alcohol, or when you use legal or illegal drugs, toxic cardiomyopathy will always be lurking from a dark corner. It's well worth expanding on this condition in a bit more detail.

A well-known cause of heart failure due to toxic cardiomyopathy is chemotherapy. Unfortunately, the list of patients suffering from this condition is growing. As the field of oncology is developing and improving, doctors are becoming better and much more skilled at detecting tumors. The incidences of these tumors are increasing—hence more and more chemotherapy is used today than ever before. Some of these chemotherapy compounds might have a disastrous side effect on our heart muscle.

The doctors are fully aware of these side effects. This is why at the start of certain chemotherapy courses, they insist on performing an ultrasound examination of the patient's heart to assess the health of all heart functions. The overall performance of the heart muscle must be normal and healthy.

Did you know that there are certain mutations that can affect the function of the heart muscle? They are unfortunately also responsible for heart failure. You may have heard about these mutations—we call them familial cardiomyopathy, while most folks refer to them as "heart conditions that just run in the family."

It's not uncommon to see a patient arrive at the hospital with a poor functioning heart, while their coronary arteries, valves and heart rhythm are perfectly normal. If all the tests and examinations can't point the doctors into one of the above mentioned cardiomyopathies, it's safe to say that we're dealing with an idiopathic cardiomyopathy. *Idiopathic* is an obscure medical term, you might think. And you would be right, idiopathic is a fancy way for doctors to say, "We don't know what caused your disease." So an idiopathic cardiomyopathy is a puzzle for medical science—the cause of this condition is yet to be discovered. No apparent cause means we have to be careful how we approach it. We simply don't know what causal factors have led toward the degradation of the heart function and how it will develop in the future. Medical science has come very far, yet there are still many mysteries to be solved.

Speaking of mysteries, myocarditis is something that can cripple any of us. Why do some people have it and others don't? Honestly, it's impossible to say; we simply don't know yet. The same goes for infections. Some people happily walk around carrying dangerous bacteria and viruses in their body without a single cough or a hiccup. Others can get incredibly ill, such as our next protagonist.

Peter is a perfectly average twenty-two-year-old university student who is getting ready for a "rather heavy" night out with friends. It's Thursday evening, and the approaching spring decorates the city with a false sense of warmth and radiant sunshine. In other words, Belgium can be quite beautiful (and cold) during spring time. Peter can't be bothered with a thick and "lame" winter jacket, so he simply hops onto his bicycle wearing just his pants and a thin T-shirt. The night is young, and the boys squeeze every ounce of fun out of it.

Fast-forward to 4:30 in the morning—time to go home and get some well-deserved sleep. The notoriously unpredictable Belgian weather decides to show Peter the middle finger and proceeds to drench his highly intoxicated persona with a relentless cold shower. Peter is cycling back home, doing his best to maintain a fragile balance, avoiding tenacious obstacles along the way. It's a gargantuan challenge, but he's hellbent on returning home in one piece, no matter the cost.

Like so many Belgian students, Peter manages just a few hours of sleep after that rough Thursday night. Right now, it's not the time to ponder the consequences of his actions just yet. Even the monstrous hangover will have to wait. Now, it's time to spend the weekend at Mom and Dad's place to regain his strength and maybe sleep a bit longer. Peter shuffles his numb body to the station, jumps into a train, and waits until the moment he can finally ring the doorbell of the house where he grew up.

As his mother opens the door, she immediately notices that Peter had a "pretty rough night." He looks exhausted and fully spent. There's even a slight lingering coughing that he just can't shake off. When Mom finds out that he has been cycling without a jacket—drenched with cold rain, she gives him the full rant only a mother can. She warns him that his reckless behavior is a magnet for potential diseases. Moms are truly the same in every country of the world!

Peter is slowly digesting Mom's words as the hangover shoots bolts of lightning through his head. He wisely decides not to argue—it's time to call it a day and melt into the sofa. The next day, what do you know? Mom turned out to be right! Peter is shivering and burning up with fever. The only good news—the hangover has finally released its iron grip and moved on to find another victim. It takes five days before the fever subsides—yet the feeling of guilt is still lingering inside Peter's consciousness. Goddamnit, mom was right! It's time for him to man up and focus on university studies. For a few weeks he's going to all classes—diligently avoiding wild parties with friends.

As Peter plows through his courses, he begins to notice a strange feeling of fatigue descending onto him. Every day he cycles to all classes, wears his winter coat, and diligently carries all his books in his backpack. However, every time he arrives to class, he needs to catch a breath and relax. During the evenings the same scenario is playing out—he even goes to bed much earlier just to combat the strange fatigue that just can't seem to leave him alone.

Is it time to worry? After all, he's just twenty-two years old and in perfect physical condition. Surely it's merely the exhausting school schedule that's slowly getting under his skin—draining his energy in the process, right? Three weeks pass and the same strange fatigue is still here with him—now even preventing Peter from concentrating on his studies. As the new symptoms show up out of nowhere (swollen feet and lack of appetite), his parents ring the alarm bells.

Peter decides to visit his family physician for a quick check-up. As the doctor is listening to his lungs, he notices something very peculiar—Peter's heart is racing so fast and violently, it seems it wants to break through his chest cavity. This is normal for a professional athlete who just crossed the finish line, yet Peter is sitting on the examination table, gingerly breathing in and out. The doctor is perplexed. He doesn't know what's causing the heart issues, but it's definitely something that needs further examination.

He orders Peter to visit the emergency room of a large hospital and demand an urgent cardiological examination. In the hospital, the emergency doctor reluctantly calls Peter inside, mumbling to himself, "What kind of amateur doctor orders a healthy twenty-two-year-old guy to go for an urgent cardiological examination at 8:00 p.m.?" The young man doesn't even have any prior heart conditions! What the hell is going on here?

The emergency doctor finally examines Peter and agrees that something is terribly wrong. Sure, the kid is not looking like a fresh, crispy pickle, but heart disease? Come on! Surely it has to be just pneumonia, or issues with his gastro-intestinal plumbing. Students are famous for treating their bodies like human dumpsters. The doctor asks Peter a few questions about his symptoms before proceeding with the clinical examination and a series of tests. And what do you know? There is something wrong with the heart after all. For starters, the blood pressure is way too low to be remotely considered normal. The doctor takes a blood sample and proceeds with an electrocardiogram (examination of the electrical signals of the heart itself).

As the results come in, the doctor cannot help but gasp in disbelief! The blood sample indicates a disturbance of all organ systems, and the electrocardiogram is looking way too abnormal. Perhaps the family physician was right after all? It's time to call a colleague cardiologist! He arrives armed with an ultrasound device, ready for further investigation. From the very first ultrasound image it's clear that Peter's heart is in big trouble. Although it's contracting at a rate of more than one hundred times per minute, there's barely any blood circulation taking place. Peter's ejection fraction should be around 60 percent (if you remember, this is an indicator of how much blood the heart pumps with every contraction), yet now it's just barely hitting 15 percent. Without exaggeration, Peter is standing with one foot in the grave.

Peter shares his story of the past few weeks. He tells the doctors everything—the infection, fatigue, and the lot. Based on the lack of prior heart conditions, the doctors immediately think myocarditis. An infection has caused damage to his heart muscle, affecting the heart function as a result. The only way to be sure is to run more tests.

Unfortunately for Peter, time is a luxury he doesn't have—he can last a few hours, but no longer. No matter the final diagnosis, his body desperately needs oxygenated blood. The organs are screaming in agony as we speak. As the doctors are helping Peter through this hellish night, the nurse is asking us to leave his hospital room for now. Let's move on to the next part of our book. We'll check back with Peter later on and see how he's holding up. I promise!

Heart Failure

Our heart is nothing more than a very efficient pump. When the pumping function of our heart decreases, we call it *heart failure*. Remember the normal ejection fraction of 60 percent? When we are looking at 30 percent, it's a valid reason to start worrying. In general, we can classify heart failure into two groups—acute and chronic.

Acute heart failure is definitely serious—the pumping function immediately fails after initial damage to the heart. One of the best examples of this condition is when a myocardial infarction leads to loss of a large portion of the heart muscle. Another example would be heart muscle inflammation—myocarditis. Honestly it would be better to face Mike Tyson in a boxing ring than to face acute heart failure head on. Yes, it's that serious! Without an immediate urgent treatment, the patient is in big trouble.

In other cases, some time may pass since the initial damage occurred, all the way until the failure of the pumping function of the heart becomes noticeable. The best example would be valvular cardiomyopathy—issues with the heart valves. It takes time before we see considerable damage. Another example is a *small myocardial infarction*. Overall, it takes time before heart failure develops into something seriously life-threatening. Very often, symptoms can fly under the radar, and for a while, the patient won't notice the severity of the situation. Welcome to *chronic heart failure*!

In many cases, the patient gets through the phase of acute heart failure with a heart that recovered from the acute, damaging event. Unfortunately, there are also cases where a patient only partially recovers from an acute heart failure, only to end up in the category of a chronic one. Whatever the cause of a declining heart function may be, the progression of chronic heart failure is always the same: the heart will begin to grow and expand.

This happens simply because our heart needs to develop a better, much more violent pumping force. To do so the heart uses a trick it has up its sleeve. You see, when you stretch a muscle, it can then create a greater force. So in chronic heart failure the ventricles will dilate, stretching the muscle fibers and squeezing with every force they have left. Every cause has an effect. The bigger ventricles will exert higher pressure on the muscle wall; hence this section will need to become a bit more beefed up, leading to hypertrophy of the heart. From cheetah to lion, remember? As time goes on, what happens to the heart muscle itself?

As it expands, more and more connective tissue is needed between the heart muscle cells. Over time, this will of course lead toward a significantly worse performance of our heart muscle. How does the heart deal with this inconvenience? You're right! It becomes even more beefed up—expanding and enlarging itself as a result. It's a vicious cycle of expansion and enlargement that eventually leads toward heart failure. Sadly, this process can take years to metastasize and usually remains unnoticed by the patients as the symptoms are quite vague.

Chronic heart failure

Normal heart   **Heart Failure**

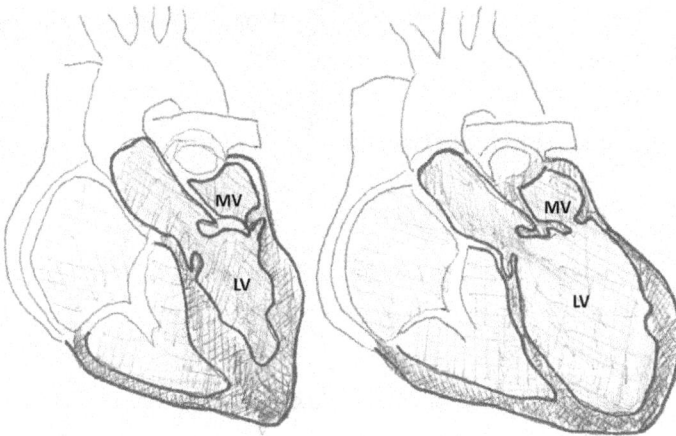

Figure 11.
Whatever the cause of heart failure is, the reaction of the heart is quite the same. The left ventricle (LV) starts to dilate and the muscle mass increases. In later stages the dilatation of the ventricle becomes more pronounced relative to the hypertrophy of the muscle. This gives the impression of a thinner wall while the total muscle mass far exceeds that of a normal, non-dilated ventricle.

When we mention the symptoms of heart failure, we need to remember that a poorly functioning heart will affect pretty much every single organ in your body. The blood doesn't circulate properly—causing congestion in the veins of the pulmonary and systemic circulation. One of the tell-tale signs to watch for is swollen ankles. You see, as the blood flow slows down, liquid will ooze out of your tiny blood vessels and start accumulating in your body's tissues. Gravity pulls on this "free wandering liquid"; hence the ankles swell first.

This liquid can also wreak havoc on your lungs. When this liquid becomes a permanent unwelcome guest in your lungs, you'll start noticing shortness of breath. Let's follow the blood flow even further. As the heart is failing to deliver the much-needed oxygenated blood to your muscles, you'll feel your physical capacity diminishing before your eyes.

Lifting heavy objects and performing enduring physical activity will feel like a losing battle. As if the ankles, lungs, and muscles haven't suffered enough, let's not forget about the kidneys. These guys need plenty of blood in order to function properly. When your heart is doing a poor job, your kidneys will become sluggish and over time might even require dialysis.

Please don't treat your body like a dumpster! The sooner you seek medical treatment, the better. With the right approach, the progression of heart failure can be stopped or at least slowed down. What can happen when you ignore these warnings? At some point, your heart simply can't handle the vicious cycle of endless expansion and enlargement, and before you realize what has happened, terminal heart failure will come knocking on your door. As you keep ignoring the obvious painful reminders, there will come a stage when even medication is powerless to help you. Remember, a big heart only works in romantic movies—not in real medicine! It helps to listen to the symptoms that your body is so desperately trying to communicate to you.

If by now you're sitting at the edge of your seat, nervously biting your fingernails, let's explore the treatment for heart failure. After all, the art of medicine has come a long way over the past decades. Yes, there's still light at the end of the tunnel!

CHAPTER 3

TREATMENT OF ACUTE AND CHRONIC HEART FAILURE

WHEN WE EXAMINE EVERY SITUATION FROM THE MEDical point of view, there are in fact several phases of treating heart failure. Fortunately, you can already begin with the first one—prevention. Remember, it's always better to prevent a disease than to cure it. Let's get off the couch, put down that glazed donut, beer or cigarette and discover how to regain our personal power.

Phase one is called *primary prevention*. Although during this phase there is nothing suspicious yet, it's important to keep our body in a normal and healthy condition. You don't have to be a rocket scientist to know the importance of a healthy diet and regular exercise, as well as strict avoidance of tobacco. And if you fancy a drink, go ahead and have one, but keep this habit in moderation. In short, this is plain old common sense. It's even taught to young kids in primary school.

Remember, you and you alone are responsible for this. In a world where sedentary lifestyle and a disgustingly unhealthy dumpster diet is the defacto norm, nobody can ever force you to improve yourself. Body shame yourself into taking action, or ask your friends to motivate you into improving your life. Now put down this book and go for a walk, run, or clean your home. You'll instantly feel better and much more revitalized! Your heart will thank you in the long run. Now that you're rediscovering your inner-Rocky Balboa, let's move on.

Even with a normal healthy lifestyle, it's not possible to prevent all heart diseases. As you remember Peter's story, there are infections that can wreak havoc on your heart muscle. We have to keep in mind that these illnesses can attack anyone—even healthy and active people. This is of course not a reason to give up on improving your health, simply because healthy people will have a much higher chance of getting through a nasty myocarditis in one piece (even to the point of making a full recovery).

As you see, primary prevention can be summed up as becoming healthier and stronger and cultivating a much tougher, "hairy chested" body that will withstand anything nature throws at it far better. This applies not only to withstanding heart diseases, but all diseases. Start today and don't delay! The simple truth is, you are much more powerful than you realize.

Now that you're glowing with optimism, I refrain from my role as a personal trainer and let's examine what secondary prevention is all about. This is simply preventing symptoms or potential damage caused by an illness. There can always be something lurking in the darkness that you're blissfully unaware of. A classic example is hypertension—high blood pressure. You don't generally feel that something is "off," and you simply continue living as you always had. Having high blood pressure for a day or two will not hurt you at all, but when it continues for years and years, your blood vessels will get damaged. One day, you can wake up to a cerebral infarction or a nasty case of constricted arteries.

Another case of such criminal body negligence is dealing with intestinal polyps. These little guys can occur in our intestines and remain benign for years. One day, however, they can turn into full-blown colon cancer. When you hear about medical screening programs, you can immediately think of secondary prevention measures. There are tests, screenings, and blood examinations that can help spot the risks of serious illnesses in their early (and much more preventable) stage. This is something your family doctor is quite familiar with—don't be a stranger in their office!

What about the secondary prevention for heart diseases? In this case we'll be checking your blood pressure and cholesterol levels in the blood. These tests can tell us a great deal about how you're treating (or neglecting) your heart and arteries. Controlling your blood pressure and keeping cholesterol levels low is the best way to stay out of nasty heart troubles in the long run. On the other hand, neglecting the first and second prevention stages can have dire consequences—a full-blown failing heart. What happens then?

We're left with no other choice but to move to the third and final prevention step—the heart disease is already noticeable and we want to do our very best to prevent it from getting out of control. Enter tertiary prevention. During this step we'll be focusing on alleviating the symptoms and treating the illness itself. One of the examples is of course implantation of an artificial heart pump. It's worth noticing that this is merely one of the last steps in treating heart failure—we'll make sure to expand on this step later on. Again, it's important to make a clear distinction between treating the underlying heart disease and heart failure itself.

For example, when heart failure is caused by constriction of the coronary arteries, it's quite self-explanatory that we will need to focus on the coronary arteries in the first place. This means opting for a stent or a bypass surgery. Remember Jan, the construction worker? First thing the doctors did in the hospital was opening his constricted artery.

However, it's self-explanatory that we need to address heart failure as well. The treatment of heart failure is not dependent on the cause of this heart failure. It sounds a bit complicated, so let's break it down. Imagine that the heart failure is caused by either the constriction of the

Coronary artery bypass grafting (CABG)

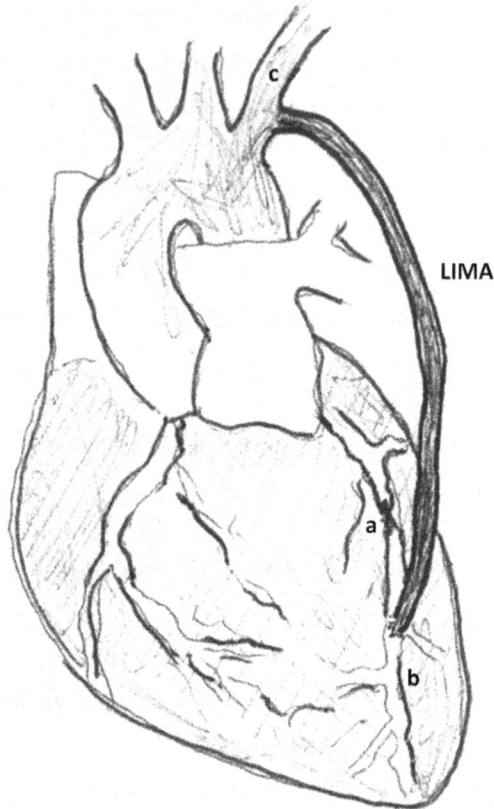

Figure 12.
During bypass surgery (CABG), the coronary stenosis (a) is literally bypassed. The left internal mammary artery (LIMA), an artery you can live without, is harvested from the chest wall and surgically connected to the diseased coronary artery (b) behind the stenosis. The blood now flows from the subclavian artery (c) through the LIMA to your coronary artery, bypassing the stenosis.

coronary arteries or some toxic substance (two different causes). We can perform a bypass surgery for the constricted coronary arteries, but the heart failure will not miraculously disappear after the surgery. So we have to treat it. If chemotherapy triggered the heart failure, we cannot undo the chemotherapy anymore. We only treat the heart failure. In this case the treatment for heart failure would look very similar to the

Percutaneous Coronary Intervention (PCI)

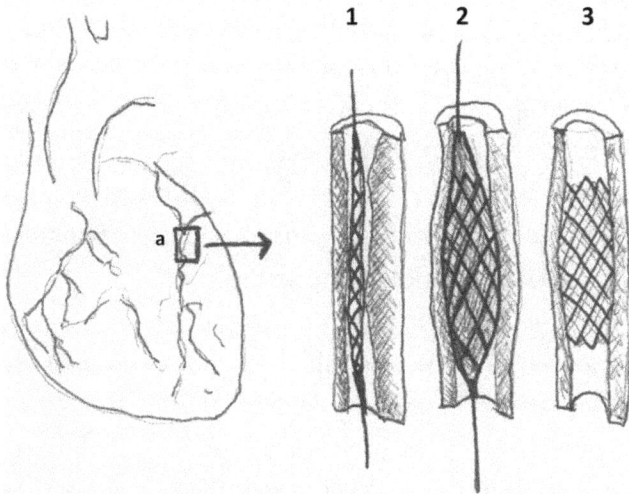

Figure 13.
During a percutaneous coronary intervention (PCI) a thin wire is inserted into the bloodstream. Under fluoroscopic guidance the wire passes the coronary stenosis (a). Over this wire a stent is brought to the stenotic part of the coronary artery (1). The stent is collapsed on a balloon. Once in the correct position, the balloon is inflated and the stent expands, dilating the stenotic coronary artery (2). At the end of the procedure the wire is removed and the stent remains in the coronary artery, preventing restenosis (3)

heart failure treatment of the patient with the constricted coronary arteries. If we truly want to understand the treatment of heart failure even better, let's divide it again into acute and chronic.

ACUTE HEART FAILURE
This form of heart failure occurs immediately after the catastrophic event that affected the heart muscle. The best example would be the inflammation of the heart muscle or a myocardial infarction. It's self-explanatory that we will focus primarily on alleviating the cause, as well as ensuring proper blood flow to our entire body, but how exactly?

In this example we'll use medication. Remember when we talked about all the nerves and hormones regulating the heart? They tell our heart how fast (and how powerfully) it needs to pump the blood around at any given moment. Today we can use several medications to activate these systems that regulate our heart function—artificially directing our heart to pump faster and with a bit more power and oomph. We have to be very careful though. You see, these medications only perform a supporting function, and we certainly cannot use them for a long period of time! We'll stop once the cause of acute heart failure has been solved and the heart function is improving.

After all, in such a short period of time, the vicious circle of heart failure has not yet been activated fully. This means the heart muscle can rejoice at the prospect of a speedy recovery. The other side is unfortunately also possible—some acute heart failure cases can be so severe that the heart stops pumping blood all together. You may have heard about it in films and TV series. It's called a *cardiac arrest*.

As you may have guessed, we'll need to take immediate drastic measures and start administering a heart massage technique that you may also have heard about. It's called cardiopulmonary resuscitation—CPR. If you have ever seen CPR in action (even on TV), the method is very straightforward. We use a compressing motion on the patient's chest in order to administer external pressure on the atriums and ventricles of the heart. By compressing the heart's chambers, you push the blood out. The valves will make sure it goes in the right direction. When you relieve the pressure in between compressions, the elastic tissue in the heart recoils and the heart fills up with blood for the next compression. These external compressions are sufficient to pump blood through the body and prevent damage to vital organs. No oxygen = no life, remember?

While the patient is kept alive, we can try to use medication to help the heart restart its natural pumping action all by itself. Sometimes, though, even this is not enough. There are cases when we need to use gargantuan amounts of medications just to keep the heart going— naturally, this can be extremely dangerous. In this case we'll opt for an artificial heart pump and let the machine take over the heart function entirely. These kinds of devices are designed so they can be quickly connected to the patient's blood circulation. The most famous of these devices is the ECMO device. Will cover this big shot later in more detail. It was this kind of device that saved Michael after his near-death experience on the golf course. Speaking of very sick patients, this reminds me to check back with Peter!

You remember Peter, right? Our unfortunate reckless hero is now suffering from inflammation of his heart muscle. Last time we saw him, he was still in the emergency room—his heart was having a truly bad time, to say the least.

Just a few weeks ago Peter's heart was still functioning normally. Now he's crippled by acute heart failure. Life can be a bitter and cruel hag! The ER doctors determined that his heart function is quite poor—there's in fact very little blood currently reaching his vital organs. These organs are now literally gasping for a breath. The doctors don't waste time and administer intravenous medication, combined with an oxygen mask.

The IV drip is currently spreading norepinephrine across Peter's body. This substance resembles adrenaline that's produced naturally by our adrenal glands. Now Peter's arteries contract and his heart can pump with a bit more force. As the blood pressure rises, his organs can finally rejoice at the sight of more oxygenated blood. Let's not forget that this is just a temporary measure that allows us to help our unfortunate patient until he makes a full recovery.

Peter's heart—an old-school combustion engine that's on the brink of shutting down—is now receiving a short boost of nitrous oxide. This will keep the engine from stalling permanently, but at what cost? We can't overdo it without risking serious damage.

In Peter's case, we're dealing with extremely low blood pressure—his organs are dancing with potential and complete failure. Doctors will need to do more to save his life. For now we have yet again overstayed our welcome in Peter's room. The doctor's angry look says enough—we need to leave.

Instead of endlessly wandering the corridors of the hospital, we can check in with Jan—the construction worker. As you remember, Jan's long career of unhealthy lifestyle has eventually brought him to a full-blown myocardial infarction. It was thunder on a sunny day, right there on the job site. That myocardial infarction made Jan's pre-existing heart failure acutely worse. In the medical field we call this "acute on chronic heart failure."

Currently Jan was also hooked up to the IV drip filled with norepinephrine. This helped his old and battered heart pump enough blood during his coronary intervention. Once the coronary artery was back open, the doctors drastically lowered the dose of medication. After a few more hours Jan didn't require any more norepinephrine at all.

We haven't heard from Michael yet. Remember how our golf player suffered the same myocardial infarction? In his case it was the worst-case scenario of myocardial infarction—a full-blown cardiac arrest! It took a complete resuscitation procedure with heart massage and adrenaline just to give Michael a fighting chance to hold on to life itself.

Adrenaline, the big brother of norepinephrine, is much more powerful, and it's the real deal! After it's coursing through the body, the heart will pump even harder and the arteries will constrict even further. If you remember, in Michael's case, even this extreme step wasn't enough, so the doctors did what was necessary and connected him to a full-blown artificial heart machine. For now we can't linger in Michael's room too long.

As we walk through the hospital halls, what other medications can we use aside from adrenaline and norepinephrine? There's dobutamine, milrinone, and a plethora of other exotic-sounding medications, each with their very own distinctive functions. Don't fear, and don't panic! We'll not cover all of these interesting substances in this book. It should be fun to read, right? Not a medical textbook. So now let's examine what we can do for patients with chronic heart failure.

CHRONIC HEART FAILURE

It's time to take a breather and let your nerves calm down from the previous section. After all, chronic heart failure treatment is fundamentally different from acute heart failure treatment. You see, we're dealing with already existing heart muscle damage here. Oftentimes this damage is unfortunately irreversible. Let's imagine that the vicious circle of heart failure has cursed our patient with this irreversible damage. What happens next?

Do you remember how the remodeling process works? This is when our ventricles dilate and become beefed up and thicken with newly formed tissue. Our patient may be blissfully unaware of this, but our eagle eye has spotted the problem. Time to roll up our sleeves and see what we can do.

The most logical treatment in this case is to prevent this progressive process of remodeling—or maybe even reverse it in the case we are blessed with the possibility to do it. Again, we know that there's damage to the heart muscle that we can't repair, yet maybe we can manage to reverse the vicious circle of progressive remodeling that the heart is currently so preoccupied with.

Enter medication! In general, the three most important medications we can rely on when chronic heart failure emerges from the shadows are beta blockers, ACE inhibitors, and diuretics. Let's take a moment to explain in detail how these three amigos work and what they do. Not only is this extremely interesting, but maybe someday this knowledge will help you better understand why you have to take all these pills.

Beta blockers slow down the heart rate and the force of the heart contractions. I can already hear the sound of grinding gears in your brain. Yes, you read it correctly—slow down the heart function. You see, although it sounds contrary to what you may expect from the normal process of treating heart failure, the point here is to help the heart work itself out of the vicious cycle of remodeling. Beta blockers manage to do just that.

It's worth noting that it took some time before the use of beta blockers became common practice. In the past we didn't prescribe them to people with heart failure; however, over time doctors saw the light and agreed that this medication is in fact extremely effective. Today beta blockers are one of the cornerstones of the effective treatment of heart failure, simply because they help to break the vicious cycle of remodeling. Let's move on to ACE inhibitors.

Before digging into the medical terminology, let's meet angiotensin. This is a peculiar hormone that increases our blood pressure and helps to strengthen the connective tissue of our heart muscle. Angiotensin is made from angiotensinogen in our body. Angiotensinogen doesn't have any effect, but once converted to angiotensin, the show begins. Your blood pressure increases, and connective tissue is formed. When it comes to angiotensin converting enzyme, ACE, this is nothing more than one of the proteins that helps convert angiotensinogen to angiotensin. Naturally, as you may have guessed, if we can block ACE with medication, no angiotensin is formed, and our blood pressure becomes lower and our heart muscle less stiff. Although these ACE inhibitors are fantastic medications, they do have a very important side effect.

ACE inhibitors reduce our kidney function. This is definitely not something trivial, and in some cases we have to resort toward a complete suspension of the use of this effective medication, as our kidney function is just too important to brush aside. Besides, when a patient is suffering from a serious stage of heart failure, the kidneys are already stressed to the maximum. Moreover in the final stages of heart failure the blood pressure can be too low to tolerate the added blood pressure lowering effect of ACE inhibitors. There would simply not be enough blood pressure left to circulate the blood through your body. Remember, a lack of oxygenated blood is a surefire way to rack up irreversible damage to our internal organs. Let's move on to the third medication: diuretics.

No doubt you have heard about diuretics. Sometimes we jokingly call them *water pills*. Yes, as you may have guessed, diuretics ensure that excess moisture is removed from the body. Aside from frequent toilet visits, diuretics prevent our ventricles from stretching out too much. When it comes to our patients, these diuretics help to relieve the symptoms of heart failure. As you may remember from previous chapters, patients in the late stages of heart failure often suffer from excess moisture that accumulates in their ankles but also in and around the lungs. This is exactly what diuretics help to remove, proving their effectiveness in today's medicine.

Now that you know how beta blockers, ACE inhibitors, and diuretics work, it's worth noting that there are a plethora of other medications that benefit patients with heart failure. Some of these medications can keep the symptoms of progressive heart failure under control. This can be well into the late years of a patient's life—giving people the possibility to live a happy life even while nursing a heavy heart condition.

When heart failure takes a nasty turn and morphs into something more life-threatening, even the best and newest medications become powerless to help. Fortunately, this is not the time to give up the fight and hang our scrubs on a coat hanger! It simply means we need to pick up the pace and start exploring other options.

If you're around sixty and you're feeling a bit dreary about your age, don't despair just yet! Did you know that according to medicine, you can still qualify to be called a strapping young lad or lady? This makes you a potential candidate for a full-on heart replacement. You see, when a patient dies of severe brain damage, they can become an organ donor. You may not know this, but the heart, lungs, liver, kidney, pancreas, and even the entire gastrointestinal tract can be used to save the lives of several people who qualify to become suitable receivers.

The very first heart transplant was performed by none other than Christiaan Bernard in 1967 in South Africa. We have come a long way since then. As of today there are thousands of heart transplants taking place all over the world. Naturally, as you may imagine, there's a chronic shortage of donor hearts. For example, in a country like Belgium, there are only twenty-five to thirty organ donors for every one million people. If you think these numbers are extreme, consider that out of this small group of donors only five to seven are actual heart donors.

Belgium is home to a respectable eleven million people. This brings the availability of donor hearts to a tiny fifty-five to seventy-seven units each year. To say that there are simply not enough hearts to go around for every patient is a massive understatement. On the other hand, not everyone who is in end-stage heart failure will be a potential receiver of a heart transplantation. Why? There are several important factors that we need to account for. When a patient suffers from severe diabetes or has a tumor, this can unfortunately lead to complications after a heart transplant. Also, a psychological assessment is necessary to see whether the patient has the ability to cope with the responsibilities that come with a heart transplant. As there are only a limited number of hearts available, we have the responsibility to use them wisely. That may exclude some heart failure patients from a heart transplant entirely. Again, let's not give up hope, but simply explore other options!

In the past fifteen years we have witnessed an upcoming trend—the long-term heart pump. You see, an artificial heart pump can be manufactured in greater numbers and is much more readily available than a donor heart. When a heart transplant candidate has to grind their teeth and wait for many agonizingly long months or even years until a viable donor shows up, the artificial heart pump is ready to go immediately, ready to save lives at a moment's notice. This is an exciting field of expertise that we'll make sure to cover later on. Now, it's time to check back with our friend Jan.

Right now, our hard-working guy pulled through at the hospital, and today he's finally allowed to go home for the first time. As you may remember, Jan is still quite a young guy, yet today he'll meet his new best friend—the pharmacist. As you remember, Jan has been through a hell of an ordeal at the hospital. Lucky for him, he's alive! Today he's picking up a prescription for new medications that he'll be taking daily. The menu consists of cholesterol and blood pressure–lowering drugs, as well as one beta blocker and one ACE inhibitor. Bottoms up!

Every morning and every evening the traumatic events at the hospital should remind Jan to be vigilant with the medication schedule. After all, his life depends on these very medications. However, as you may imagine, the perfect world where people take their medication on time and on schedule only exists in the pages of novels and on TV screens. Yes, after a traumatic event scares the living hell out of a patient, they will be extremely vigilant with their medication schedule. With time, however, the attention span will become a bit more wobbly. It's quite self-explanatory what kind of further self-inflicted damage this attitude can invoke over time.

Right now, Jan is deciphering the facial expression of his pharmacist—perplexed and mildly confused, to say the least. You see, just a week ago he didn't even know that there was a doctor who specialized in every body part—but he's learning fast!

Do you remember Lucas? He's the patient who was born with a transposition of the great arteries. Thanks to the early life-saving surgery, he's alive and well! He even became a dad for the first time. Lucas is no stranger to doctors and pharmacists. Due to his complicated health condition, he has been a frequent visitor to hospitals and pharmacies. He knows that aside from a cardiologist (heart specialist), there are nephrologists (who specialize in kidneys) and even gastroenterologists (who are looking after people's gastrointestinal tract). Lucas's quite unique condition requires him to undergo frequent tests and screenings—eventually directing him toward proper medications that make his life longer and more fulfilled.

Lucas is taking medication that treats his heart failure. Coincidentally, he's also taking a medication similar to what Jan is picking up from the pharmacy right now. Both Jan and Lucas are young lads through doctors' eyes. They both require similar medications, yet the progression of their heart diseases will look quite different. We know that Jan's coronary artery has been opened up—allowing ample blood flow to continue supplying his vital organs. Now it's time to put on his big-boy pants and improve his life. If he keeps on track, it will lead him away from the grim reality of a potential terminal heart failure.

Lucas's story is, unfortunately, quite different. As you remember, for the last twenty-seven years his heart has been working like an athlete! His heart pumps blood throughout his entire body using the wrong ventricle that's absolutely not made for this job. He's using a bicycle pump on a car tire. It works, but the tool is just not made for the job. In this case Lucas needs to diligently follow his medication schedule—his life depends on it! But unfortunately it probably will become a losing battle in the long run.

Every patient is unique and, in their own way, extremely fascinating. As doctors we are doing our best to save as many patients as we physically can. But ultimately every one of us also needs to take personal responsibility. So do your bit of primary prevention, or in other words—live healthy! Don't be a stranger to your family doctor (secondary prevention) and if you have to be treated (tertiary prevention); take your pills! There's nothing more precious than a human life and the time given to us to enjoy it.

CHAPTER 4

MECHANICAL
HEART PUMPS

AS YOU REMEMBER, OUR HEART IS JUST A BLOOD PUMP.
It uses pressure to direct the flow of blood in just one direction—supplying every part of our body with rich, oxygenated blood. Take a look at the stuff around your house, and you'll find pumps everywhere—from coffee machines and swimming pools to bicycle pumps and compressors. The function is always the same: pressurize water or air and send it in one direction, from place A to place B. If the tech-savvy brains already designed these common pumps, that means making artificial heart pumps shouldn't be such a big deal, right?

Unfortunately for us, things are not always that simple. Remember the chapter about blood? This is not *just* a liquid. It's also home to so many other cells and substances, all of which our body desperately needs to stay alive. The classic rotor (the spinning part of a pump) could easily act as a makeshift meat grinder and seriously damage our blood. This is why we need to tread very carefully and design a perfect pump that will treat our blood (and all the substances in it) with the gentlest touch possible.

You see, our blood is a living organ. Throughout our evolution, our heart, blood vessels, and blood became perfectly tuned to one another, allowing the perfect balance for blood circulation throughout our body. In other words, our blood, heart, and blood vessels are made as one perfectly functioning unity of components—all designed to deliver blood to our organs in the most safe and efficient way possible.

An artificial blood pump is a technological clockwork of metals and plastics. Sometimes it can generate high pressures and flows that far exceed the natural pressure of our heart. These seemingly unsolvable issues have united small armies of doctors and engineers to eventually come up with the viable solutions that we see today. Naturally, it took a long time before doctors took the risk of using these pumps in the practice of heart surgery. Something as vital as an artificial heart must be the pinnacle of reliability. Swiss watches, eat your heart out!

As we dive into this fascinating topic and examine all the modern technological wizardry that is the artificial heart pump, it's important to make some distinctions between long-term and short-term pumps. Short-term pumps allow the patient to stay comfortably alive for days (and even weeks) until another solution can be provided.

When it comes to long-term pumps, these amazing machines are much more permanent and can help a patient to live for months and even years. No artificial heart pump is ideal. There are, however, some very important basic requirements that a good artificial heart pump should fulfill.

Artificial Heart Pump's Hippocratic Oath

1. I shall do no harm to the patient's blood.

Our blood is a living, breathing organism packed with its own quite sophisticated defense mechanisms. After all, if you accidently cut your skin, your blood will sense this tissue damage and will set in motion several processes to help us patch up this gaping wound as fast as possible. We owe our life to this amazing function of our blood. It not only keeps our body's borders intact, but it also protects us from unwelcome guests. It simply knows when a foreign object is interfering with our body, and it goes out of its way to repel this intruder. It may be a bacteria, the stinger of a bee, an arrow tip that accidently landed in your thigh, or, in the case of this book, an artificial heart pump.

Yes, you heard it correctly. A mechanical heart pump is a collection of metals and plastics. Our blood doesn't like it one bit! You see, the blood loves to come into contact with the familiar tissue of our arteries and veins—this is our blood's home. When the blood suddenly finds itself flowing through some odd piece of plastic tubing or, even worse, a metallic rotor, it will rightfully start to revolt!

The blood will kick into action and will do its very best to form a protective clot around the unwelcome intruder that suddenly wreaks havoc inside the warm and familiar pipeline of our blood vessels. Luckily, we have medications that can anticoagulate blood—limiting this natural defense mechanism. Despite the blood thinners the risk of clot formation always lurks around. Engineers work tirelessly to reduce the probability of this happening to 0 percent, but of course nothing is truly as perfect as our own natural heart. However, we have come a long way, and the latest pumps require far fewer anticoagulants than older models and have very low rates of blood clots developing inside the pump. If you're curious, the correct name for this condition is *pump thrombosis* (thrombosis = blood clot).

Now that we have solved the clotting issue, let's talk about *shear stress*. It takes a certain amount of force to push our blood through our entire system of blood vessels. When the blood works its way through an artificial heart pump, sliding along the surface of the moving parts, it encounters a certain mechanical resistance that's called *shear stress*. This shear stress is also present between the inner lining of our blood vessels and our blood itself, and it's a pretty normal phenomenon. The laws of physics always apply.

A normal, healthy patient will have relatively low shear stress, but when a patient is suffering from calcified deposits inside the blood vessels, this shear stress will be higher. Unfortunately, the same phenomenon can be seen when we're dealing with constricted and calcified heart valves. When the shear stress is too high, our red blood cells will scream in agony and are torn apart. This is called *hemolysis*, and it's definitely no joke! So a good heart pump has to produce a low shear stress!

As you still remember, our red blood cells love to transport oxygen. By now you may imagine what can happen to the red blood cells during hemolysis. That's right, our oxygen transportation mechanism begins to suffer! As if this isn't bad enough, during hemolysis, the protein that helps bind oxygen to our red blood cells (called *hemoglobin*) is released by the cracked red blood cells and starts roaming the vast spaces of our blood circulatory system.

For every action, there's an equal reaction! When our blood plasma becomes rich with this hemoglobin, our kidneys can filter it out and restore the natural balance. A small amount of hemoglobin is a piece of cake to filter out. The troubles start when this amount is too damn high. It can overwhelm the kidneys to the point of a complete kidney shutdown. You have been warned!

If you notice that your urine becomes red (and in later stages of hemolysis even a dark brown color that resembles cola), it's safe to say that you need to drop everything and head to the hospital right away. The free-wandering hemoglobin has reached your kidneys!

As you see, shear stress is no joke. It can do some serious damage to your blood and eventually your vital organs. Sometimes, though, this shear stress can have a completely different impact on our blood plate-lets. They suddenly activate and start going to work creating tiny blood clots. These tiny blood clots can start hanging out in different places throughout our body. If they are found obstructing arteries near the vital organs, they will naturally wreak havoc on the blood circulation, starving our vital organs of oxygenated blood. In other cases these tiny clots can start to form inside the artificial heart pump itself. There they might interfere with the spinning of the rotor.

By now we can safely say that a good artificial blood pump has to be designed (and even over-engineered) in such a way that it doesn't damage our blood! Naturally, today we can test every new pump design using artificial setups of blood vessels where real blood is doing its work.

Aside from these complex experiments, engineers can also run computer simulations, sniffing out every potential nook and cranny inside a heart pump. We can now accurately search for areas where shear stress is lingering too high—waiting to cause potential damage to our blood.

The engineers and doctors tirelessly poke their noses into every new pump design, trying to determine the best possible candidate for the job. The holy grail of this work is an artificial heart pump that is 100 percent hemocompatible—fit for human blood. After all, the greatest risks of future complications are associated with this hemocompatibility. We need to get it right!

We already know that our blood doesn't like any foreign object. Although our blood acts like a hairy-chested bouncer with a face chiseled out of a slab of granite, it also has a hidden soft side and can quickly rack up serious damage when confronted with an artificial blood pump. Naturally, this means the materials of the pump must never cause any form of toxicity.

2. I shall be compact.

If we're dealing with serious life-and-death cases, we can afford to sustain a patient's life using heavy and bulky machines, such as the ECMO. This philosophy goes straight out the window whenever we are talking about long-term artificial heart pumps. You see, these light and compact pumps need to work tirelessly for months and even years. In the ideal case, the patient should have full and unrestricted mobility while their heart pump is happily buzzing away, working its magic.

Nowadays you don't see anyone walking the streets dragging a full-size ECMO machine with them, do you? We're very fortunate that technology has come a long way. The majority of long-term heart pumps are so tiny that they can even fit into the pericardium (the connective tissue that surrounds our heart muscle). The patient is perfectly mobile and can enjoy a second chance at life. This wasn't always the case.

In the past, these pumps were a lot bulkier. During surgery, we needed to create some extra space inside the abdominal cavity (right under the diaphragm) to provide them with a permanent home. Luckily these days are over. Today only babies and toddlers cannot physically accommodate a full-scale long-term heart pump. Instead, they receive a pump that lives on the exterior, while only the necessary tubes enter the chest cavity and eventually end up connected to the heart. Life always finds a way!

3. I shall be technically perfect.

When it comes to long-term heart pumps, we are literally dealing with matters of life and death. If we can expect our washing machine to break after fifteen to twenty years, we can't say the same about an artificial heart pump. Also, it isn't that simple to fix a broken part when it is buried deep in the chest of a patient. We can't cut any corners and compromise a fail-proof design in any way. After all, the patient's life is at stake here.

Now that we finally understand all three criteria that make a long-term artificial pump a viable heart replacement, we cannot help but marvel at today's technical achievements! Now we have had our five minutes of daydreaming, let's see what all the buzz is about when it comes to short-term heart pumps.

SHORT-TERM HEART PUMPS

As you remember, short-term pumps are designed to help a patient for a few days and sometimes even weeks. The very first short-term pump was used back in 1953 by Dr. Gibbon, and it worked for an impressive forty-five minutes during an open-heart surgery. The machine took over the function of the heart of an eighteen-year-old female patient while the surgeons worked tirelessly to repair her heart defect. To put it all into context for you, during the times when radios had massive vacuum tubes sticking out of them, this new technology was already there to help save lives. Without any exaggeration, this is pretty damn impressive!

During the 1950s and 1960s these amazing machines were further refined, to the point of becoming a true medical revolution in the art of heart surgery. Aside from simply pumping blood, these machines could also take over the function of the lungs—oxygenating the blood as well as removing carbon dioxide on the other end. If you remember the beginning of this book, we talked very briefly about these so-called heart-lung machines. Back in the old days, these machines were used mainly during heart surgery—never exceeding twelve hours of permanent use. Some minds in the medical community were seriously considering the vast possibilities of these short-term heart pump machines—mainly as a means of effective help for patients with acute heart failure. As the machine could theoretically take over the heart and lung function—in this case for a period longer than twelve hours—it would give doctors time to treat the heart condition and save the patient! However, it would take another few years until this dream became a reality.

In the 1970s the first-ever ECMO machine kicked open the doors of technical innovation! If you're curious, ECMO is simply an acronym for *extracorporeal membrane oxygenation*. Although it sounds a bit complicated, it simply means that the oxygenation process takes place outside of the body (extracorporeal) by means of a membrane—some people call it an artificial lung. This membrane is the key part of transferring oxygen to the blood and removing the carbon dioxide.

As the oxygen is deposited, the ECMO pressurizes the blood and sends it back into the patient's body, ensuring that every vital organ can now enjoy a steady supply of freshly oxygenated blood. The machine can handle a few liters of blood every minute without as much as a hiccup! It goes without saying that in a healthy body, our heart and lungs are responsible for these important functions. Now we can help a patient with a failing heart—the ECMO works tirelessly to keep them alive.

We can boldly say without exaggeration that over the past decades, the ECMO has helped to save countless lives worldwide. The doctors

Extracorporeal Membrane Oxygenation (ECMO)

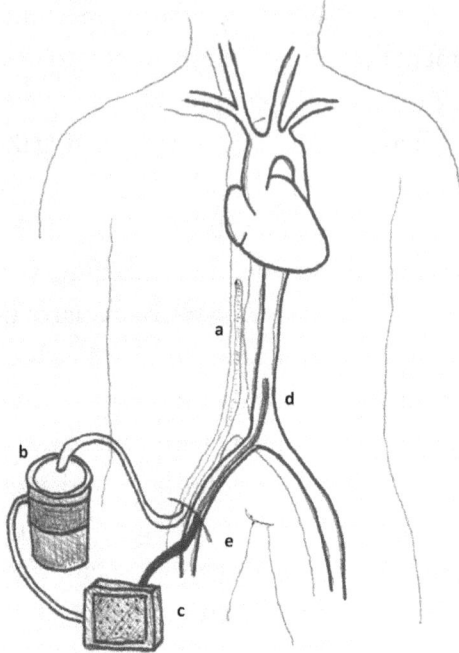

Figure 14.
An ECMO device can take over the entire function of the heart and lungs. A cannula (venous cannula) in the vena cava inferior (a) will drain the venous blood to the machine. There it enters a pump (b) that pressurizes the blood and sends is off to the oxygenator (c) that removes the CO_2 and adds oxygen to the blood. This oxygen rich blood then enters the systemic circulation through a cannula (arterial cannula) in the descending aorta (d).
Blood is drained from the venous side and given back to the arterial part of the systemic circulation. As such the ECMO renders the heart and lungs obsolete and bypasses the pulmonary circulation.
Both cannulas are inserted in the artery and vein in the groin using a small incision (e) and are advanced into their correct position in the blood vessels.

swear by these machines and use them quite frequently; however, they do have a sizable drawback—the patient is completely immobilized and in effect chained to the hospital bed. Why?

First of all, the ECMO is a large, bulky machine that, just like a loyal spouse, never leaves the side of the patient's hospital bed. There's a large tube that's connected to the patient's femoral vein. It feeds blood into the ECMO machine, while the oxygen-rich blood re-enters the patient's body via the femoral artery. These two tubes enter your body in the groin, where the femoral vein and artery live—making unrestricted mobility pretty much impossible.

The strategic location of the femoral vein and artery makes it easy for the surgeon to connect the patient to the ECMO in the shortest amount of time—in many cases saving the patient's life as a result. Check out Figure 9 in the very first chapter. It will help you refresh your memory.

As you can see, this ECMO device isn't a long-term solution for heart failure. There are just too many downsides for long-term use. The patient is literally chained to the hospital bed, the groin area might get infected, and there is the risk of bleeding as well. There are just too many factors that can complicate the patient's situation, and this is exactly why the ECMO (even today) can only be considered as a transitional solution toward something better and much more comfortable.

So why use ECMO at all? Well, when we're dealing with a patient who's suffering from extremely life-threatening acute heart failure, the ECMO becomes a worthy candidate. You see, in just a few minutes, we have the ability to transfer the complete heart and lung function to the machine— in essence saving the patient's life. No other machine can do that! It can be done in a hospital, but in some rare cases it can happen on the street as well. Nothing is impossible! So ECMO is a powerful tool, but only to get through the toughest and roughest phase of extreme heart failure.

Fast-forward two weeks, and as the patient's condition becomes stable and the heart has a chance to recover and resume its normal function, the use of the ECMO can be stopped. There are, of course, cases when the heart is too weak to recover. But let's not give up hope just yet! This simply means we will need to explore other alternatives—a heart transplantation or a long-term heart pump.

When we're treating patients with acute heart failure, it's important to note that not all of them will have issues with their lungs. Therefore, not everyone will require a machine that also takes care of the lung function. Do you remember the two blood circulatory systems? The systemic circulation takes care of the needs of all of our organs, while the pulmonary circulation only handles the lungs. This simply means that patients who only require assistance with their systemic circulation won't require a machine to help oxygenate their blood. What does this mean for the design of our artificial heart pump?

You're spot on! It means we can make the design much simpler, due to the lack of oxygenation features. This translates to a smoother operation, less resistance, and less potential damage to the patient's blood. Sounds like a win-win situation, doesn't it? Yet, not everything is as easy as it seems.

You see, connecting this device to the circulatory system of the patient is not as simple as the ECMO. We are pretty much cut off from using the femoral veins and arteries in the patient's groin. We would end up pumping the oxygen-poor blood from the veins directly into the patient's arteries, resulting in too little oxygen in the arterial blood. This is definitely something we want to avoid. Instead, we need to divert the already oxygen-rich blood (that passed through the patient's lungs) to our pump, pressurize it, and send it to the arteries of the systemic circulation. Unfortunately, this blood that just came from the lungs lives in our left atrium and ventricle, buried deep in the chest of the patient, a place difficult to reach in short notice during acute heart failure. So doctors and engineers literally began thinking outside the box (of left atrium and ventricle).

This concept gave birth to *counter pulsation*. In this procedure, a narrow balloon-like apparatus is implanted into the aorta (after the blood flow passes the arteries that nourish our brain). Just like any normal balloon, it inflates and deflates. As the balloon inflates, it pushes the blood to our cerebral vessels and back toward our heart. As you may have guessed, this means our brain and heart receive more blood flow.

The balloon's mechanism is neatly synchronized to our heartbeat— as the heart goes into diastole (relaxation), the balloon is inflated. As

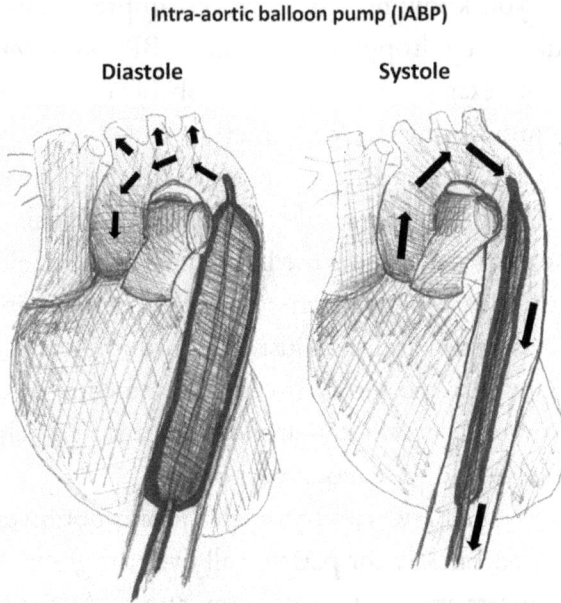

Figure 15.
The intra-aortic balloon pump is inserted into the aorta from the femoral artery.
During diastole it will inflate, pushing blood into the supra-aortic vessels and the coronary arteries, increasing perfusion to the brain and heart.
During systole it will deflate, reducing pressure in the descending aorta and facilitating the ejection of blood out of the left ventricle.
Black arrows indicating blood flow during diastole and systole in the aorta.

the heart muscle contracts (systole), the balloon deflates—effectively lessening the drag on the blood flow. This is quite beneficial to a patient with a weak heart, as this deflation mechanism, in essence, creates a suction force as the blood is sucked into the aorta. This entire mechanism is implanted through the femoral artery in the groin area. There's an external control unit that uses helium for the inflation and deflation action that's perfectly synchronized to the patient's heartbeat.

Although you may be reading about this invention for the first time, you may be surprised to learn that this system was invented back in the 1960s, and it quickly gained popularity for treating myocardial infarction.

Now that you know how it all works, impress your in-laws at Christmas dinner by dropping the name IABP (*intra-aortic balloon pump*). Without exaggeration, this was probably the most commonly used heart pump worldwide. Why exactly?

You see, it's fairly straightforward to outfit the patient with this device. The procedure is not terribly invasive, and the risks are low. As all coins have two sides, so does the IABP. Due to the small volume of just 50 ml, this device's effectiveness is indeed quite limited—at any given time it can push and suck just a minute amount of blood out of the heart and into the aorta. As if this wasn't enough, our patient needs to have a steady heartbeat that allows for perfect synchronization between the heart and the balloon pump.

In the past the IABP was pretty much the only option doctors had at their disposal. Luckily for patients all over the globe, the tireless minds of engineers and doctors are never at rest. As the options for heart pumps become more plentiful, we have seen a steady decrease of the use of the IAPB over the years. Ready to look at other cool new developments?

Over the years, as we have mercilessly dispatched the boundaries of technical possibilities, we came up with new and exciting technical solutions that made the pumps smaller and more compact. How compact exactly? How about just a few millimeters? That's right, today we can achieve a respectable blood flow of a few liters per minute using nothing more than a tiny pump with a rotor the size of just a few millimeters. These dimensions allow for greater flexibility and maneuverability. The pump becomes so tiny it can be mounted on a catheter that we use to navigate the blood vessels. We can now implant these catheter-mounted devices directly through the blood vessels that are easily reachable (the femoral or axillary artery). As you may imagine, this greatly simplifies surgical procedures for the doctors and greatly reduces risks for the patient.

These modern space-age short-term heart pumps are the latest and greatest in the field of modern medical science. The surgeon can use the

Catheter-mounted pump

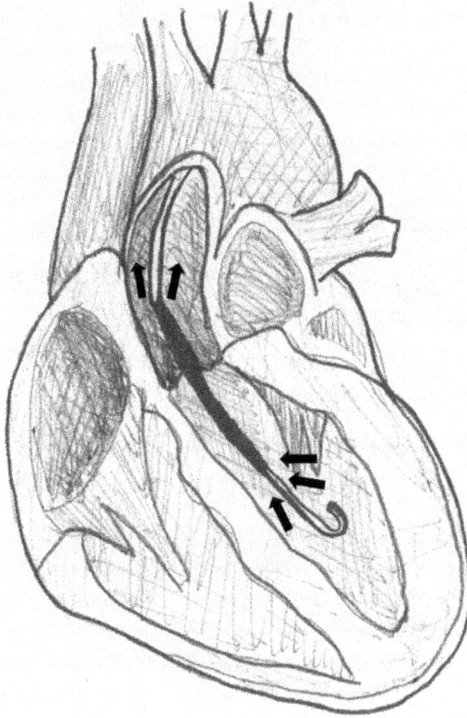

Figure 16.
The catheter mounted pump is inserted into the left ventricle either from a peripheral artery (femoral or axillary artery) or direct from the aorta.
The blood enters the pump near its tip and is pushed out at the end of the pump, which is situated in the aorta.
Black arrows indicating blood flow generated by the catheter-mounted pump.

femoral artery to push this device into the correct position—passing the aorta and ending up all the way in the left ventricle. The very tip of the pump is nestled inside the left ventricle, while the bottom sits in the aorta. That's right, the pump passes through the aortic valve. The aortic valve even plays an essential role in allowing the pump to work properly. As the pump sucks blood at its tip in the left ventricle and ejects it into the aorta, the valve will prevent the blood from going back into the ventricle. From the moment the pump kicks into action, a patient with acute heart failure can immediately experience its effect—improved blood circulation without the need for further blood oxygenation. In short, the oxygen-rich blood that returns from the lungs is pumped straight into the systemic circulation, providing a life-saving flow of blood to the patient's body. Sound complicated? Take a look at Figure 16, and it all becomes much clearer.

You may be surprised to hear that these pumps have already existed for more than twenty years. However, today they are becoming quite popular for treating patients suffering from acute heart failure. We are seeing that these new catheter-mounted pumps are replacing the balloon pumps and their bulkier brother, the ECMO. Today these tiny devices can even be implanted through the axillary artery (the large blood vessels that pass through our shoulder). If you forgot about this part of our anatomy, you can always check Figure 9 in Chapter 1.

As you can imagine, working with such a small device connected to the axillary artery gives our patient much-needed mobility! After all, when you're chained to the hospital bed, hooked up to the ECMO, this mobility becomes fiction. The tubes in the groin make walking around or even sitting up straight impossible. Totally different story with a catheter-mounted pump that only has a very thin tube exiting the skin at your armpit. Now our patient is free to roam around and contemplate how lucky they are at the prospect of having a second chance at life. Aside from this amazing benefit, it's important to keep in mind that the catheter-mounted pump can remain operational for a lot longer than the bulky ECMO machine. Now we can help the patient build a strategy such as a heart transplantation or a more rugged long-term heart pump. Speaking of long-term heart pumps . . .

LONG-TERM HEART PUMPS

In life, we must always remain optimistic! Sometimes, though, we need to ask ourselves difficult questions, such as, "What happens if the patient's heart function does not recover completely?" Again, let's not fall into despair, but simply explore other options—the use of a

Pulsatile LVAD

Diastole

Systole

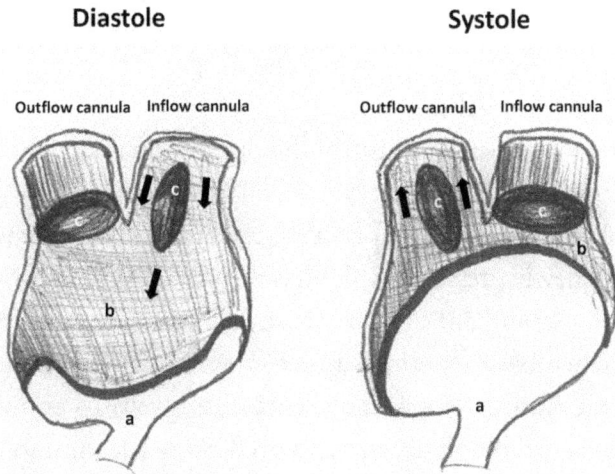

Outflow cannula   Inflow cannula

Outflow cannula   Inflow cannula

Figure 17.

During diastole, the gas chamber (a) is empty, blood flows in the artificial ventricle (b). One-way valves (c) prevent blood from leaking back from the outflow cannula (connected to the aorta) in the artificial ventricle.

During systole, , the gas chamber (a) is filled, blood flows out the artificial ventricle(b). One-way valves (c) prevent blood from going back into the inflow cannula (connected to the ventricle).

Black arrows indicating blood flow during diastole and systole in the device.

long-term heart pump. How can we best define *long term*? In our case we're talking about supporting the patient's blood circulation for many years—reliably and continuously.

Back in the 1960s, as the world indulged itself in rock and roll and dubious amounts of mind-altering substances, doctors and engineers were already hard at work—kicking open the doors of technological innovation in the medical field. We could already perform surgical procedures on heart valves and coronary arteries, but unfortunately, when the heart muscle itself became completely depleted, even the best doctors became powerless.

There was a clear need to design something that would replace an ill heart in its entirety. How in the name of science could we pull it off?

The human mind started searching for answers that produced some very interesting options. One of them was building a completely artificial heart—a machine that used membranes and hollow chambers to imitate the natural function of our heart. The membrane sat between two chambers—one for blood and one for gas. The entire unit was powered by an external console.

As you can see, the mechanism of this pump is quite straightforward. When the gas inflates one part of the chamber, the other part (that contains blood) becomes compressed—essentially creating a pumping action. This newly pressurized blood is then ready to move onward. If you weren't sleeping during your physics lessons back in high school, you may remember that liquids love to travel down the path of least resistance. Our heart solves this problem by using valves—ensuring that highly pressurized blood doesn't end up flowing back into our veins. This artificial heart essentially used a similar system.

Although this new machine worked, it was still quite bulky and difficult to implant into the patient's chest cavity. Aside from this, there were reliability issues—oftentimes with catastrophic effects. For example, there were issues with tears in the membranes, as well as blood clots that formed on the valves. So in practice, these artificial hearts were only used for a short period of time—no more than two years. They were only a temporary solution to keep the patient alive until a donor heart became available. Now that we have covered the internal mechanism, what about the external system?

Unfortunately, the problems didn't stop there either. You see, the bulky compressor needed to provide the pumping action was a nightmare to drag around. The sheer level of noise that the damn thing made would even give an astronaut's suit a run for its money. The technology was truly in its infancy, and there was definitely room for improvement. Back to the drawing board!

The much-needed breakthrough came with the arrival of electromagnetic compression plates. Gas went out the window, and together with it, the loud and bulky compressor unit. Now the patient was finally relieved of all the heavy metal that needed to be dragged around wherever they went. Though this problem was solved, we were still dealing with the risks of leaky membranes and blood clots inside the valves.

This design is called the first generation of artificial heart pumps. We call these *pulsatile devices* simply because they all use the same principle of pumping action. An internal artificial ventricle is filled with blood and pushed empty. A patient outfitted with this type of pump will still feel a recognizable pulse at their wrist. Over the years we have seen several designs and improvements of these units. Doctors used them quite frequently during the 1980s and 1990s, saving many lives in the process.

In the beginning of the 2000s, we witnessed the biggest breakthrough in the evolution of heart pumps. For the first time ever, we were able to propel blood using an impeller mechanism instead of membranes. From now on, we'll call these devices *rotary blood pumps*. The biggest advantage of using this design is, of course, the complete elimination of valves and membranes (that made the pulsatile devices bulky and unreliable).

Although this natural evolution seemed like a logical step forward, there was plenty of trial and error along the way. For a long time doctors thought that a human body would not be able to handle such a heart pump. Why exactly? You see, since we're working with an impeller, we need to crank it up to very high speeds if we want to have the slightest chance of achieving the needed pressure and blood flow inside the patient's circulatory system. We're talking about a few thousand revolutions per minute going even up to 20,000 rpm in some smaller pumps!

No wonder the doctors were skeptical. Think about it: not only would our blood need to pass this high-speed impeller, but it also needed to squeeze itself through very narrow spaces (we are talking about a millimeter or two here) between the stationary pump body and the moving parts. We naturally assumed that our blood (and all the important vital substances that it transports) would be greatly harmed by this shake-up. Luckily, with the right design of the pump, our blood handles it quite well.

The next logical question on the agenda was, "How well will our body handle the non-pulsatile continuous blood flow?" We truly have to marvel at our own anatomy, simply because this also doesn't appear to be such a vital issue as we previously suspected. You see, when our blood travels to the far ends of our vascular system, the pulsatile effect of the heartbeat is almost non-existent. So in the smallest arteries of a healthy person, the blood flow is already non-pulsatile. As long as our blood is sufficiently pressurized, oxygenated, and flowing well, we're good to go! Let's dive into the mechanics for a second.

As you now know, the first-generation pumps used a gas compressor to inflate and deflate a special membrane or an electromagnetically driven compression plate. So how does the impeller mechanism work? Just like any other electric motor, the rotating action is achieved with the help of magnetic fields. The new generation of heart pumps all use this electromagnetic motor to drive the impeller, pressurize the blood, and send it in one direction to wherever it's needed inside our body. As you see, we went from pulsatile pumps to full-on magnetic motor pumps—or as we like to call them in medical terms, second-generation heart pumps.

It's important to mention that today, even the third-generation heart pumps all use the same propulsion mechanism. The natural question is, of course, "What's the difference between the second and third generation of heart pumps?" The answer is *friction*. Look at the moving parts inside a car engine. They all require ample lubrication. Without oil, the moving parts of your engine would destroy themselves in mere minutes. The same laws of physics apply to the impeller of the heart pump, except this vital machinery cannot just be lubricated at random. We need to ensure maximum durability in order to give the patient years of carefree use.

The second-generation heart pumps used rugged and reliable ceramic bearings to keep the rotor in place. Although it sounds counterintuitive, ceramic materials are tougher than steel, and over time they show less wear and tear. Unfortunately, nothing is perfect. With time, as these ceramic bearings start to wear down, our blood starts to form clots in these areas. This increases the overall risk to the health of our patients.

Enter the third generation! Now the impeller is held in place using magnetism—effectively floating on magnetic bearings. This means the impeller never makes contact with the pump housing and shows very little wear over long periods of use. Naturally, this design decreases the risk of blood clot formation, which is music to the patients' ears. You may not know this, but the system of magnetic levitation is used all over the world inside submarines. No friction between the moving parts means no noise! But then again, why should the military have all the fun? It's better to use such amazing technology in medicine.

Now you know how artificial heart pumps work; it's time to see how they are implanted into the patient's body. This will be a very interesting chapter.

CHAPTER 5

HEART PUMP IMPLANTATION

ALTHOUGH YOU MAY BE EXCITED TO DIVE STRAIGHT in, let's take a moment to make an important distinction between short-term and long-term heart pumps. You see, both devices are very different and require a totally unique approach, both in strategy and the surgical procedure itself. Let's start with short-term heart pumps.

IMPLANTATION OF THE SHORT-TERM HEART PUMP

As you remember from the previous chapter, we can help our patients using three different types of short-term heart pumps.

1. ECMOs—the bulky machines that completely take over the heart and lung function. Yes, they will save your life, but at the cost of being chained to your hospital bed for a few days and sometimes even weeks.
2. Catheter-mounted pumps—they pump the blood right out of the left ventricle and send it straight into the aorta, thereby improving systemic circulation. They are small and nimble, allowing you the freedom to roam around and enjoy your second chance at life.
3. IABPs—the famous balloon-like pumps that support the left ventricle and improve systemic circulation by inflating and

deflating with every diastole and systole. These were once the absolute kings of mechanical support in acute heart failure, but their reign is now challenged by the new kids on the block.

Now it's time to wash our hands, put on the surgical gown, and get the tools ready. We're heading to the operating theater . . .

ECMO

Aside from the obvious drawback (of decreased mobility of the patient), the ECMO system can be connected with very limited means. No wonder it's the most preferred system we use when dealing with severe acute heart failure. When we are dealing with a patient who is dying, every second counts! The doctors start by making an incision in the groin area and implanting two tubes, one in the femoral artery and one in the femoral vein. How does it work from here? The oxygen-poor blood is sucked out of the femoral vein of the patient and flows directly into the ECMO machine. Inside the machine, the blood is scrubbed of all the nasty carbon monoxide, oxygenated, pressurized, and sent back through the femoral artery into the patient's bloodstream. Remember, we're dealing with an ill heart that's simply too weak to work properly, a heart so weak that even the pulmonary circulation can't be served. No blood going to the lungs means no oxygenation, and oxygen is life! This is why the ECMO machine takes over and keeps our patient alive.

Let's follow the bloodstream. Now, as the oxygenated and pressurized blood enters the systemic circulation through the femoral artery, it can easily flow to all the organs and ensure every single organ can profit from fresh oxygen. If you remember Figure 9 in Chapter 1, you'll see something strange: inside the arteries, the blood is actually traveling in the wrong direction! If you look closely, you'll see the blood is flowing in the following direction:

1. Starting from the femoral artery
2. Going to the aorta

3. Flowing to the head of the patient

Don't panic, this is perfectly acceptable! You see, there are no one-way valves inside our arteries. This means as long as oxygenated blood is present inside the intricate network of our arteries, it will inevitably find its path to all our organs and deliver the oxygen wherever it's needed most.

Now imagine the following situation: your patient has just collapsed, and we need to work as fast as humanly possible. What now? Without wasting a second, we make a small incision in the groin area and implant the tubes. This can also be done using a so-called puncture technique. In the worst-case scenario (a full-blown resuscitation), we can have the ECMO up and running in just minutes. The beauty of the entire procedure is that we don't require any special tools—we can focus solely on shaving off the crucial few seconds that make the difference between life and death. It's worth mentioning that other short-term heart pumps will require some special equipment to guide the proper placement of the device. Currently, as our patient requires urgent help, we don't have this luxury.

Getting back to our ECMO, it's up and running. This wonderful machine can circulate a respectable five liters of blood every minute. This is definitely enough to sustain the life functions of our patient for now. Even if our patient's heart has stopped completely, the ECMO will keep their alive.

The ECMO is an amazing machine that helps patients who are suffering from acute heart failure. Without a word of exaggeration, we can safely say that this machine has saved countless lives over the years. But wait, doesn't every surgical procedure have its risks? Yes! So are there any risks associated with the use of ECMO? Short answer, yes.

You see, we are working with tubes that are implanted into the femoral vein and artery. Take the tube that goes into the femoral artery, for example. It's just a tiny bit smaller than the femoral artery itself. As you remember, the femoral arteries provide blood to our legs. You can already guess what can happen to the patient's leg if the femoral artery is invaded by a tube of the ECMO machine—the leg can experience a shortage of oxygenated blood. Up to 30 percent of ECMO-assisted patients experienced leg ischemia (oxygen deprivation of the leg) in the past.

Luckily, this issue was largely solved by adding a second (smaller) tube to the leg. When the ECMO is up and running and the patient is out of the immediate danger zone, we can afford ourselves the luxury of tuning the patient's situation. We can now make a smaller incision right under the main tube and implant a leg cannula (a smaller tube) into the femoral artery. Now the patient's leg will have access to as much oxygenated blood as it requires.

Once our patient is stable (and the leg is provided with oxygenated blood), we can still run into a few issues. You see, sometimes the ECMO can start to counteract the patient's heart itself. It sounds a bit counterintuitive, so let's explore this situation a bit further. As the ECMO machine is keeping our patient on life support, it provides ample blood flow and pressure inside the cardiovascular system—providing every organ with oxygenated blood. If the patient's heart is recovering, it tries to resume its natural function of systole and diastole (pumping action), and it will try to pump the blood through the aortic valve. As you now know, the blood flow is coming from a different direction—the ECMO itself literally counteracts the heart's natural one-way blood flow.

In the ideal situation, the patient is alive, the heart can slowly recover and the artificial blood flow of the ECMO can be weaned off. In this case, as the ECMO blood flow becomes less important, the heart can start to resume its normal function—playing solo violin on the stage that is the patient's body. This is great news! The ECMO can finally retire.

What about those other cases when the heart is simply too ill to resume its normal function? In this case the ECMO blood flow will be pushing against the aortic valve of the patient. The valve will remain closed, and we will be inevitably dealing with static blood that

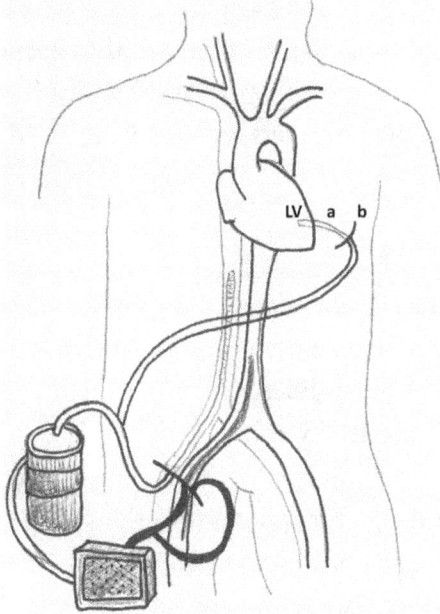

**Extracorporeal Membrane Oxygenation (ECMO)
with transapical venting and leg cannula**

Figure 18.
An ECMO device taking over the function of heart and lungs. The left ventricle (LV) is unloaded by a cannula (a) inserted through a small incision (b) at the level of the apex of the ventricle.

accumulates inside the left ventricle. You may already guess what can happen next—stale blood can start forming clots inside the left ventricle, and with time, the heart function can deteriorate further. It's time to take urgent and drastic action. The life of our patient is hanging by a thread . . .

We urgently need to relieve the left ventricle of the lazy, stale blood. Luckily, we can insert a small tube directly into the left ventricle and drain this blood directly into the ECMO. This means, of course, an additional incision in the chest of the patient, which is not ideal, so we sought new ways of dealing with this stale blood in the left ventricle. In the past few years, we have been using catheter-mounted pumps to prevent blood from accumulating inside the left ventricle. These pumps help propel this lazy blood over the aortic valve and into the systemic circulation. With time, we have learned to perform all of these procedures with great speed and agility.

Today it's possible to help the patients in the emergency room and even right on the street where they collapsed with a case of acute heart failure. During emergencies, every second counts. This means we have to be ready at a moment's notice. I'm happy to report that we are!

CATHETER PUMPS

Now that you have a better understanding of ECMO, the next type of heart pump will be easier to understand. You see, the catheter-mounted pumps have a few peculiar differences. In medicine, size does matter! Contrary to the thick, bulky tubes of the ECMO, today's catheter pumps are so tiny, they can entirely fit inside our arteries. The entire assembly, down to the motor and pump body, is designed to be as slim and non-invasive as possible. Pretty cool, right?

We can now manipulate the entire device, guiding it through the arteries and precisely positioning it where it's needed—inside the patient's body. The inflow part of the pump passes the aortic valve and ends up directly in the left ventricle. The business end of the pump, a small motor that lives inside a thin tube (where blood is ejected under pressure), remains inside the aorta. As you may imagine, if we wish to work with this heart pump, your aortic valve (the valve between your left ventricle and aorta) has to work like a Swiss watch. If the valve has an important leakage, there is no barrier between the inflow and outflow part of the pump, and blood is just pumped in a tiny circle from outflow to inflow. When the valve is constricted, we simply cannot push this pump assembly over the valve to its correct position. The same goes for your arteries. When you have heavily calcified and constricted arteries, we cannot maneuver the damn thing even close to your heart.

Let's assume that our patient's condition allows us to use the catheter pump, and we are happily assisting just the left ventricle. As you remember from previous chapters, the right ventricle needs to provide ample blood to our pulmonary arteries and lungs. What happens if the heart is functioning poorly, and the right ventricle is not up to the task? You may have already guessed it: in this case there won't be enough blood arriving inside the left ventricle. The catheter pump will not be able to save our patient in that case. Bring in the ECMO! This means that catheter pumps are, in essence, only assisting the left-sided heart function of the patient. You might think that this implies that only a few patients can benefit from these catheter-mounted pumps. Well, not exactly. Most myocardial infarctions impair the function of the left ventricle much more than that of the right ventricle. And let's not forget the left ventricle is the bodybuilder doing all the heavy lifting, pushing the blood at greater pressures through your whole body. In the case of a heart issue, the left side will much sooner need assistance than the right ventricle. So, the catheter-mounted pumps do deserve a place in our surgical toolkit. How do we go about implanting this amazing device?

Just like with the ECMO, we will use the thick femoral artery for this procedure. Contrary to the ECMO, this femoral artery is just the beginning of our long journey through the anatomy of our patient's cardiovascular system. When we need to end up nestled between the left ventricle and aorta, we need to wiggle and maneuver our pump through the femoral artery and the aorta. The procedure is not for the faint-hearted (pun intended). Luckily, the surgeons are quite skilled at this procedure.

Sometimes, though, we can use a shortcut—the axillary artery (located in your armpit). If you feel like cheating, take a look at Figure 9 in Chapter 1 again. Although this artery is a bit more difficult to reach, you may have already guessed why we would opt to use it. It's all a matter of mobility. When we use the axillary artery, the patient is free to move and walk around at their leisure. Having a small tube in the femoral artery near the groin area will definitely complicate this mobility by a great deal. I hear your brain rattle, "Why not always use the axillary artery?" Well, it is harder to reach, and it lies so deep that in order to have a good access point for the catheter-mounted pump, we even need to extend the vessel with a graft. None of this is needed in the femoral artery. Again, it all comes down to time. If we need to assist the systemic circulation immediately (in a resuscitation), we have to go to the femoral artery. Is the patient's heart failing but we think it can keep going for another thirty minutes? Let's go and dig toward that axillary artery then.

Let's assume for a moment that we have found the artery and we are ready to proceed. How do we go about maneuvering our catheter pump into the correct position? For this procedure we will need specialized X-ray machines that usually live in large, well-equipped operation rooms. Remember the ECMO? We can connect this machine to our patient in less than ten minutes, and any hospital room will do. No need for fancy X-ray machines. When it comes to our current case (especially when we are using the deeply tucked-away axillary artery), we will definitely need more time! The catheter pump needs to be slid, wiggled, and pushed into the perfect position inside the left ventricle. Our eyes cannot see through the patient's skin, but the X-ray machine can, showing us every move of the pump as we push it further and further down the arteries. You may think that it's a bit of a hassle, but trust me when I say, the result is worth it!

To illustrate the best-use case for this catheter pump, it's time to check back with young patient Peter. As you remember, he's been stricken with severe myocarditis. The last time we saw him, he had been kept alive with rather high doses of medication (norepinephrine) to keep his blood pressure up. Sadly, the medication just isn't cutting it—we will have to mechanically support his heart while he's struggling to recover. Now, as we bow over his hospital bed, we must make a choice between opting for the ECMO or the catheter-mounted pump. In his case, we'll go with the catheter pump. Let's examine why!

Peter's lungs are still rock solid. He's a healthy young man and he doesn't smoke. Currently, his left ventricle is failing. Due to congestion of his lungs, we are noticing that they are filling up with some fluid. We know from experience that from the moment we hook up the catheter-mounted pump, these issues will start to decline. Back to Peter's heart for a second. We know that both his ventricles are performing poorly. Although our catheter pump will only assist his left ventricle, the right one will still have sufficient function to pump blood to his lungs.

What happens when we relive the left ventricle by use of a catheter pump? The right ventricle will experience less resistance to pump the blood over the lungs and will be able to work a lot better. For Peter, this is music to his ears. Currently his condition is somewhat stable. This gives us ample time to prepare the entire procedure. For the sake of his mobility, we'll be opting to implant the pump via the axillary artery. Let's check Peter's current report.

He's diagnosed with a severe case of myocarditis. Later on, we will need to run further tests to find the exact cause of this condition. Only then will we know in what way his condition can be treated best and maybe even reversed entirely. The million-dollar question is, "How long will it all take for his heart to recover?" Currently, time is a luxury we simply cannot afford to waste. With the help of an ECMO, Peter will only have a few days' time until we pinpoint the cause of his condition. A catheter-mounted pump will not only give him significantly more time (weeks) but will also allow him the needed mobility—he won't be chained to his hospital bed!

As we're exploring all the options for Peter, you may remember how the ECMO can counteract the heart function. Due to the high blood pressure generated by the ECMO machine, the aortic valve won't be able to open, and just like described in the previous chapter, we will be dealing with the nasty side effect of lazy blood that accumulates in the left ventricle. Let's not forget that Peter's heart was healthy just a few weeks ago. If we want to see his heart making a full recovery, it's unwise to subject him to such risks.

Our very last motivation for opting to use a catheter-mounted pump is, of course mobility. Peter will be able to move around. You may not think this is such a big deal but consider this: when you're chained to your hospital bed while connected to the ECMO, you will lose about 15 percent of your muscle mass in just your first week. For the record, it is not the ECMO to blame but the fact that you are lying in bed without moving a muscle. Patients in an artificial coma in the intensive care unit have the same experience. When a patient requires additional procedures, the body becomes even weaker. Now put down the potato chips and take a minute to appreciate the perfection that is your body. If this information comes across like a brick smashing on the side of your head, it's because it should. "Use it or lose it"! This is the motto for staying healthy all the time, even if you happen to be in a hospital for a few days.

Let's go back to Peter. He's being prepped for surgery as we speak.

As he arrives in the operating theater and is administered the anesthesia cocktail to put him asleep, we are ready to proceed. We start with a small incision (no more than 5 cm) under his clavicle. Now we gain access to his axillary artery and connect the graft to it. We fire up the X-ray machine and start to navigate the catheter-mounted pump through our incision. We have finally maneuvered the catheter-mounted pump to the final destination—Peter's left ventricle. Now we can start the pump, and already after just one minute, the anesthesiologist starts to reduce the high doses of supporting medication. We are ready to wrap it up. Peter is still blissfully asleep under anesthesia. He's ready to be transferred to the intensive care unit. Tomorrow, he will wake up feeling like a fresh, crunchy pickle.

His lungs are now much less congested, and the dose of norepinephrine that's administered intravenously is now significantly reduced. We can pop the cork—the operation was a success! All of this is possible thanks to the amazing invention that is the catheter-mounted pump. Now it can take over the still poorly functioning heart and provide Peter's systemic circulation with a whopping five liters of blood every minute.

For the sake of simplicity, we have only focused on the most crucial steps of Peter's operation. It's easy to see the surgeons as absolute rock stars on the stage of the operating theater, but let's remember the efforts of the entire team of specialists who are present during the procedure to help Peter in this critical moment. This is not a solo gig, but rather an entire medical orchestra at work!

If you're really curious, during this type of operation, there are as many as seven people working hard in the operating theater: two surgeons, one anesthesiologist, two nurses, one perfusionist (who manages the pump itself) and one X-ray technician. After the operation, there's a small army of physiotherapists, nurses, and even social workers and dieticians that will help patients with a speedy recovery. Although they are not present during the surgical procedures, they are vitally important to the recovery and well-being of every single patient. As we tip our hats to them, we can proceed to the IABP pumps.

IABP

An *intra-aortic balloon pump* (IABP) is a short-term pump that's much easier to implant than the above-mentioned examples. We only require a small puncture in the groin, using the femoral artery to maneuver this device into its correct position. As you may have guessed, we also require the X-ray machine to find our path to the aorta. Although from a technical point of view this is a relatively straightforward procedure, let's keep in mind that the IABP is also the least powerful of all the short-term heart pumps in existence. All things considered, this amazing invention does deserve an honorable mention. For years it was the king of mechanical support for acute heart failure! Now let's roll up our sleeves and move on to something much more intricate.

IMPLANTATION OF LONG-TERM HEART PUMPS

The difference between the short-term pumps and long-term devices is night and day. Acute heart issues oftentimes require the use of short-term pumps. In these cases, we are literally dealing with life-and-death situations. There's very little room for error—we need to act *immediately*! Yes, the patient will be out of harm's way, but on the other hand, we only offer a temporary solution that will last days and in some cases weeks, maybe months. This is why the applications of long-term heart pumps are so different.

You see, as we are gearing up for a much more complicated and longer-lasting surgical procedure, we are aiming for at least some months and in most cases even many years of uninterrupted work—literally giving our patient a second chance at life. The long-term pump will be happily nestled inside the patient's chest cavity for a very long time. You can already imagine that removing such a pump later on will require a similarly heavy and invasive surgical procedure. Let's put away the scalpel for a second and use the sharpest tool in our arsenal—our critical thinking.

Knowing what we know now, it's important to consider that a long-term heart pump is the very last solution for our patient. In other words, we have depleted all other potential options, such as medications, heart operations tackling the underlying cause of heart failure, short-term pumps, and prayers. As we are dealing with chronic heart issues, this long-term pump will be a literal lifesaver for countless patients. But let's not forget about acute heart failure cases as well. You see, if we are dealing with a heart that's simply too weak to recover fully, we will oftentimes resort to using a long-term heart pump as a final long-term solution for the patient. In that case, the short-term device was just a tool bridging the patient to a long-term pump. Speaking of patients . . .

Sadly, not everyone can simply receive a long-term heart pump. Not that we don't want to save everyone, but we need to be realistic about the chances of having our patient survive the operation. Not only survive, but also have a chance to thrive after the operation. So what do we want to assess before going to the operating theater to implant a long-term heart pump?

Patients with severe brain damage are excluded from being viable candidates. Now imagine a patient with acute heart failure who had full-on CPR which ended in a short-term heart pump implantation (an ECMO or a catheter-mounted pump). The patient's heart simply fails to recover, so naturally, we think about a long-term heart pump. The patient is currently in an artificial coma, and it will take a while before we see them wake up, so assessing brain damage might be tricky. It might take days to a week before the patient awakes from the artificial coma. Of course, other means like a CT scan of the brain or an EEG (electro-encephalogram, a kind of ECG of the brain) can help in assessing brain damage, but until we are certain that the brain is alright, we will refrain from implanting a long-term pump. We have to be sure about the brain! If the brain damage is too extensive, a long-term heart pump implantation is pointless.

Another point of attention is the kidney function. Less-than-normal kidney function is not a problem, but full-blown kidney dialysis is not an ideal situation. Dialysis with a long-term heart pump is not impossible but definitely challenging.

Aside from these somewhat exclusive criteria, we also need to consider several important psychological factors. You see, life with a long-term heart pump requires a delicate balance between man, machine, and medication. A patient requires titanium-like discipline and adherence to a certain routine. Again, we are looking at factors that are very difficult to estimate when dealing with acute cases of heart failure. Let's exit the mental roller coaster and look at a few examples (we will call them scenarios) where we opt to implant a long-term heart pump.

It's self-explanatory that we will only cover the cases whereby a patient's heart is irreversibly failing without any chance of a swift recovery (otherwise, we would have opted for a short-term pump). But just like there are many ways to Rome, there are many ways to end-stage heart failure. So, we will encounter many different patients here, young and old, with not only heart failure but many other diseases. For example, we could have a seventy-five-year-old patient who was struck by a heart attack at the age of fifty, and from that dreadful day, the heart has been on a long journey toward complete failure. The remodeling process that we covered earlier. On the other hand, we could be dealing with a healthy twenty-five-year-old patient who ran into some nasty myocarditis just a few weeks ago. Every case is very different, and it's vitally important to make the right judgment when dealing with every unique patient. In clinical practice, we will always refer to certain terms that will point us in the right direction at every possible scenario. Speaking of medical slang, now that you have read this much already about heart pumps, let me introduce you to the term most physicians use when speaking about long-term heart pumps. We simply call them LVADs (*left ventricular assist device*). Now let's explore a few examples of different scenarios in which we use LVADs.

Scenario 1: Bridge to Transplant (BTT)

From the title alone, you may have already guessed that we are opting for an LVAD while our patient is waiting for a donor heart. As you already know from previous chapters, this grueling waiting period can run up to two years, and in some cases even longer. If we are dealing with a patient with poor heart function, we need to be extra careful at all times. You see, somewhere along the way, there's a risk that the patient's heart function will start to deteriorate to dangerous, life-threatening levels. We simply cannot afford to subject our patient to such needless suffering. Hence using a long-term pump will solve many problems during the long wait for a new donor heart.

You may not know this yet, but the very first LVADs were developed (and used) precisely for these cases. Doctors were finally confident that using this pump would be safer for the patient than lingering around with a sick heart. In the case that the LVAD started to perform poorly, we already knew that the patient had graduated as a viable candidate for an urgent heart transplant. So if the LVAD failed, an urgent heart transplantation was a way out.

As we move along the list of scenarios, I can't help but recall one of my patients. Let's meet Leo. There was nothing that would distinguish him from any other average forty-year-old man, if not for one thing—last year he was diagnosed with idiopathic cardiomyopathy. If you still remember, this is the type of heart failure where proper diagnosis is simply impossible. In other words, the heart is failing due to reasons that are unknown to modern medicine. In Leo's case, the only option we have is to symptomatically treat his condition.

As of today, it's been three months since his name was entered into the waiting list for future heart transplants. Now, it's only a matter of luck and patience. The first month was luckily quiet and uneventful. During the second month, however, Leo's condition rapidly started to deteriorate. Suddenly, the mundane task of walking up the stairs became an insurmountable obstacle. Wisely, he decided to check himself into the hospital and let the doctors run the necessary tests. As you may imagine, the situation turned out to be much more dire than previously expected—Leo's kidneys were failing as well.

The doctors did what they could to help, and with some changes in his medications, Leo was sent back home, only to return two days later with even worse symptoms—low blood pressure, shortness of breath, and full-blown kidney failure. We were back to square one, only now the kidneys were not recovering correctly, and we could not stop the prescribed medications. Leo's condition was rapidly spiraling out of control. As the onset of liver failure slowly crept into his awareness, it was time to take quick and decisive action. You may have already guessed it—Leo would receive an LVAD. The heart pump would support his left ventricle and hopefully help him out of the deadly vicious circle of total organ failure in the process. Fingers crossed!

Just five days after the LVAD implantation, Leo was a completely different man. He was already slowly walking around the hospital wing, looking forward to a full recovery. After two weeks, he was discharged from the hospital. He just needed to give his liver and kidneys some much-needed time to recover. The good news is he's back climbing stairs like never before. The bad news is his chest has become a permanent residence of the LVAD heart pump. His new mechanical guardian angel will accompany Leo wherever he may go. Let's not forget that as his condition is now stable, his name will have to be temporarily removed from the heart transplant waiting list.

Right now, Leo needs to fully recover from the heavy surgery and regain his strength. After three months he can be successfully reactivated on the waiting list. Someday in the near future he will get lucky and receive his donor heart, and hopefully he will relocate these tragic months of his life to the pages of his personal history book.

For the sake of objectivity, it's important to keep in mind that such a heart transplant (just like any heart surgery) carries risks for the patients who already live with a "steel heart." As the body adapts to the new mechanical guardian angel, it starts to grow new adhesive tissue around the heart and the heart pump. This adhesive tissue makes the heart transplantation surgery after an LVAD implantation more challenging to the surgeon. Naturally, we always keep these risks in mind and proceed with extra caution and proper care. This is, again, good and bad news for Leo. It looks like he cheated death at the cost of a more difficult and cumbersome heart transplant surgery further down the line. If that's the case, so be it. Better a bit more challenging operation down the line than dying due to heart failure today. Let's wish Leo a speedy recovery and move on.

Scenario 2: Bridge to Decision (BTD)

Imagine that you run into a serious acute heart condition. As we saw in previous chapters, acute heart failure is no joke. We need to flex our medical muscles, run all the necessary tests, and determine the cause of this ordeal. In short, we need to move mountains just to help one patient. No matter how much the doctors try to help, your heart function just fails to recover properly. In fact, the situation quickly deteriorates toward full-blown terminal heart failure. Before your incident, you were a normal average Joe with a normal, fully functioning heart. This means you had never heard of a heart transplant, let alone been on a heart transplant waiting list. What now? Put me on the list quickly! Unfortunately, as we explained before, it's not that simple. The screening to determine if you are a viable transplant candidate takes time (that our critically ill patient simply doesn't have). But don't despair. Again, the LVAD comes to the rescue! Of course, you now know that for many of these patients, a short-term pump (type ECMO or catheter-mounted pump) was the first device to pull them out of their critical state. If their heart didn't recover enough under this short-term pump, it is time for the LVAD to shine.

Now we can breathe a sigh of relief and give our patient a few months to recover. At the same time, we are free to run all the necessary tests. If our tests are successful, the patient's name can be added to the heart transplant waiting list.

Sometimes, though, things are a bit more complicated. If we happen to find a problem that we can solve, we'll always proceed to help our patient further. For example, some types of tumors require a long treatment process—during this time our patient will remain in the BTD scenario. Other times we can run into contraindications that make a heart transplant procedure impossible. Don't panic, this is not the end of the world! This simply means our patient will be living with an LVAD for the rest of their life, and they will migrate into the scenario of *destination therapy*. We'll cover it in a bit more detail later on. Now it's time to check back with Peter. He's already awake, rocking a brand-new catheter-mounted heart pump.

Peter has already spent two weeks in the hospital. His catheter-mounted pump is providing his systemic circulation a respectable five liters of blood every minute—siphoned straight out of his left ventricle. The catheter-mounted pump also provides Peter with much-needed mobility. He's free to explore the hospital on his own two feet, do some physiotherapy exercises, and even complain about the hospital food! As much as we want this story to have a happy ending, the reality can be a cruel mistress—Peter's heart is not showing any signs of recovery. His heart is as ill as the first day he arrived in the hospital.

As the doctors bow over Peter's case, it's clear that his heart will require long-term support. The conclusion is unanimous—an LVAD implantation. This option will allow him to return home and take some time to recover even more. At the same time, the doctors will be running tests and determining in what way Peter will be a potential candidate for a heart transplant.

The news is like a cinder block smashing into Peter's face. You can imagine how hard the poor guy is struggling right now, trying to make a life-altering decision. What would you do in his case? No more catheter-mounted pump, but something much more permanent. After some much-needed soul searching, hours of internet research, and conversations with people who share a similar fate, he arrives at the conclusion to go for it. Peter is quickly running out of options, so the LVAD just got a green light. Now we can breathe a sigh of relief and move on.

Scenario 3: Bridge to Candidacy (BTC)

This scenario is a tricky one. Usually, the patient meets almost all criteria needed to qualify for a heart transplant waiting list. Almost all! The majority of patients in the BTC scenario are suffering from elevated pressure in the pulmonary artery. This is a frequent side effect during heart failure—as you remember, when the left ventricle is struggling to pump blood, it will start to expand just to account for this new reality. What happens next?

The left atrioventricular valve (*mitral valve*) will fail to close properly—during every heartbeat it will be literally pulled open. As you may imagine, a poorly functioning valve will ensure that blood will start flowing in the wrong direction—from the left ventricle back into the left atrium. If we rewind the direction of the blood flow even further, we'll quickly see that this impacts our pulmonary veins as well. How exactly?

The blood that returns from our lungs should enter our left atrium with relative ease. However, this doesn't happen—the poorly functioning valve is causing chaos and refusing to close properly! As the blood returns from the left ventricle to the left atrium, there's more pressure building up in our pulmonary veins, and they quickly fill up with more blood. If the large pulmonary veins can handle this disturbance, the smaller capillaries will start to struggle and leak fluids.

This fluid happily fills up all the tiny alveoli inside our lungs. As you may know from high school anatomy, these alveoli are designed for air *only*. As months and years go by and the lungs become more and more abused and filled up with fluids, something peculiar starts to happen: the tiny blood vessels in our lungs start to build up more and more resistance. The blood is wriggling through them in the same way a sumo wrestler passes through the entrance of a subway train during rush hour in Tokyo.

All this blood flow resistance translates into a much more stressed right ventricle. It's currently huffing and puffing just to allow blood to circulate around in our (already sick) lungs. Let's keep in mind that this process is playing out across a relatively long time. This means our right ventricle has ample time to adjust itself to the new reality—little by little, it pumps harder and harder, trying to squeeze the blood through the ever-narrowing blood vessels inside our lungs. With time, the right ventricle will beef itself up and become stronger and stronger. Honestly, the situation is not looking too good at this moment!

Sometimes the pressure of the right ventricle can become so high that it can even match the pressure of our left ventricle. In normal conditions, the left ventricle handles pressure that is a whopping six times higher than our right ventricle! Let that sink in for a second. All this time, our right ventricle has been beefing itself up, just to be able to handle this new pressure. If you're curious, we call this condition *pulmonary hypertension.*

Now let's imagine that our patient is fortunate enough to receive a heart transplant. A new donor heart's right ventricle hasn't been trained to handle the monstrous pressures needed to push the blood over the lungs. In fact, the new right ventricle will be so weak that it won't be able to circulate blood across the pulmonary artery at all. A skinny toddler (right ventricle) is now trying to push against the sumo wrestler (pulmonary arteries). It simply doesn't work. The good news is that nothing is impossible. Patients with pulmonary hypertension can be helped using an LVAD. What does this look like?

When we use an LVAD, we effectively reduce the leakage of blood to the lungs over the left atrioventricular valve. Reducing the leakage means reducing the release of fluids in the alveoli and effectively cutting the driver for higher resistance in the pulmonary vessels. In many cases, after just three to six months, we can observe a noticeable improvement—the lungs don't have the same resistance as before. The result of all this mechanical wizardry? The right ventricle doesn't need to huff and puff anymore. It can function normally again.

When we finally see this reduction of pulmonary resistance taking place, this is music to the ears of our patient. Thanks to the LVAD, there are no insanely high pressures anywhere in the lungs. The right ventricle doesn't need to be a big, strong monster muscle to pump blood over the lungs. This means our patient has just become a viable candidate for a heart transplant, as an unprepared donor heart's right ventricle will be able to pump blood over the lungs.

Do you remember Lucas? Our young father is no stranger to operations. For the past thirty-two years his right ventricle has been performing the function of the big boss—powering the entire systemic circulation. If you remember, this job is usually performed by the much stronger and beefier left ventricle. Unfortunately for Lucas's congenital heart condition, the doctors solved this problem using a special operation years ago.

Although the right ventricle wasn't designed for this important job, it's been serving Lucas with nothing but loyalty for the past thirty-two years. Now it's finally starting to show its age. The right ventricle is giving Lucas a hard time—physical effort feels like a chore, and normal everyday life is becoming tough. At the age of twenty-seven, he was more or less a normal, healthy young man. Now at thirty-two, he's struggling hard. If you pass the poor guy on the street, you'll immediately notice that he's having a very bad time right now.

Swollen legs, heavy breathing, gray skin discoloration, and cold limbs—all signs are pointing toward inevitable heart failure. Although Lucas is in dire need of a new heart, he's struggling with a nasty side effect—dangerously elevated pressure in his pulmonary artery. Yes, this is a full-blown case of pulmonary hypertension in action. Let's keep in mind that Lucas has a very special heart anatomy. His left ventricle is the master of his pulmonary circulation. It's tough and beefed up and handles the new reality of elevated pulmonary resistance pretty damn well!

Currently, as Lucas is on the waiting list for being a heart transplant recipient, this is, unfortunately, a massive problem. We can't simply give him a new heart. The high pressures of his pulmonary circulation will give the new heart a very bad time. No blood will be able to flow to the lungs. The solution: Lucas is given an LVAD, and we can immediately start to see results.

First, his right ventricle will have to exert significantly less effort to service his entire systemic circulation. Second, the resistance in his lungs might start to reduce. Now we can only wish Lucas a speedy recovery. If his pulmonary resistance indeed improves, someday he will receive a new donor heart. If his pulmonary resistance remains the same, it still is much better to live with the LVAD. Why? Because he is alive! With his own heart continuing to work on its own, death would have been the next stop . . .

Let's leave Lucas so he has a chance to recover and look forward to spending more time with his family. You may not know this, but pulmonary hypertension is not the only reason we would opt to use an LVAD. Sometimes we deal with patients suffering from severe obesity. Needless to say, severe obesity is a contraindication for becoming a transplant candidate!

On the other hand, an obese patient with heart failure will have more trouble exercising and losing weight. Even with the assistance of an LVAD, some of these patients cannot shed the extra weight on their own. In these cases, we will opt for using an LVAD, as well as bariatric surgery—a procedure that reduces the stomach size and helps to lose weight over time. Of course, the operations are not combined. First you get the LVAD. Then you go on a diet and do exercise, and if all that fails, bariatric surgery might be considered. My humble advice is to try to lose the weight on your own even though it is hard!

As much sad as it is to admit, our modern trash diet and sedentary lifestyle ensure a steady stream of these issues in patients. The bottom line is take good care of yourself, physically and mentally!

Scenario 4: Destination Therapy (DT)

As you remember, not everyone makes it to the list of potential recipients of a donor heart. There are some factors that exclude patients, including age, other illnesses, and other factors. Fear not, dear reader! This simply means that an LVAD will be a wonderful option that will greatly improve your longevity and quality of life.

This scenario is reserved for patients who have arrived in their final stage of irreversible heart failure and cannot benefit from medication anymore. In short, we're talking about serious life-threatening situations. The patients in this group are usually no strangers to hospitals. In fact, most of them have already been admitted to the hospital with severe cases of heart failure a few times. Their heart failure transforms daily tasks into pure ordeals that feel like running a marathon while breathing through a straw. We are talking about the biggest group of people who are walking through life with an LVAD assisting their hearts, in what is called *destination therapy*.

Destination therapy has surpassed bridge to transplant (BTT) as the main use of long-term heart pumps. Most of the people undergoing this treatment are already a bit older than average, and aside from heart failure, they usually have some other health issues and diseases. The average DT patient is no stranger to the cardiologist, as they have had heart issues for many years. So in most cases, cardiologists had ample time to decide if this patient was a good candidate for an LVAD. There are, of course, exceptions.

For example, some patients suffer from an acute event like a massive heart attack, and the heart simply never recovers. Now, let's imagine this patient is older than seventy and the eligibility criteria for a heart transplant have been depleted. We can't afford to give up hope, so we will consider an LVAD in this case. This is the DT-scenario in action. However, let's not forget that the implantation procedure of an LVAD is, in fact, quite a heavy and stressful operation. We need to be extremely careful in our overall patient evaluation here. Writing about this topic is like walking through a minefield. We have to be careful and precise. Why?

Imagine that you are a seventy-plus-year-old person with a medical portfolio of diabetes and kidney failure. To make matters worse, you just went through a traumatizing heart attack. Without exaggeration, a full-blown MMA cage fight would have been a much more pleasant and palatable experience than what you just experienced. Think about what would happen if we subjected our patient to a heavy operation involving an LVAD. It doesn't take a specialist to estimate the high probability of a tragic outcome. Does this mean we should give up hope? Absolutely not!

In these delicate cases, we opt for short-term heart pumps. As you already know from previous chapters, these devices are much easier to implant and afford us ample time to evaluate our patient's progress. After all, we want nothing more than to see a full recovery from an acute heart failure event. In some cases, the outlook for recovery of our patient is optimistic, but the heart simply fails to recover completely. In other words, you wake up from your coma (so the brain is undamaged) with kidneys, lungs, and a liver that all work fine, but your heart is just as rubbish as on the day of your myocardial infarction. Remember Peter with his catheter pump wandering through the hospital corridors? Every organ was functioning like it was before the myocarditis, except his heart. Peter is not alone.

Many others who have a major cardiac event experience the same. During the first days after the event, all hope seems lost. Organ after organ fails (especially the lungs, kidneys, and liver), and the patient loses muscle mass being intubated and bed-bound in the intensive care unit. But after those first days, some start to recover! The million-dollar question then is, what about the culprit, what about the heart? Best-case scenario, the heart recovers as well; worst-case scenario, the heart has given up. Again, we won't lose hope, but rather start thinking about using an LVAD. We truly live in amazing times of great medical discoveries. Today people have options and access to life-saving technologies that our grandparents could only dream of. Speaking of grandparents, let's meet our next patient.

Geraldine is seventy-six years old, and she's the textbook definition of a grandma as we know it. Lately her carefree life has been brutally interrupted by a persistent pain in her chest. This pain lingers for days and makes Geraldine's life a living hell. She has no clue what exactly is causing her agony, but you and I can already guess—a myocardial infarction! You see, not every type of myocardial infarction immediately immobilizes you or causes agonizing pain that would make you sprint to the nearest emergency room.

Sometimes the signs of trouble can appear subtly, and more often than not we tend to dismiss them for something trivial such as indigestion or a case of aching muscles. This is exactly what happened in Geraldine's case. Days go by without any improvement, and reluctantly she decides to visit her family physician. Now her chest pain (although a bit more bearable) has befriended two new very odd symptoms: shortness of breath and coughing. Geraldine comes from a time when people were tough as nails, yet she decides to let her doctor help her overcome this nasty common cold. To an untrained eye, all the symptoms are pointing in this direction.

In just one week's time, Geraldine needs to look and feel impeccable for the long-awaited family reunion, so off to the doctor she goes! The family physician listens to her complaints and proceeds to examine her lungs and heart. And what do you know? All signs indeed point to a normal common cold. Out of precaution, the doctor decides to examine Geraldine's blood as well. She's an average grandma, and it's been a while since she blessed the doctor's office with her warm presence. The family physician decides to quickly fire up his ECG machine (*electrocardiogram*, a quick and non-invasive way to check a patient's heart condition) as well because her heart rate was a bit elevated. Just good practice to ensure she doesn't have an hidden arrythmia. The results are in, and suddenly the doctor's eyes almost pop out of their sockets!

We are most likely looking at a serious infarction of the anterior wall. The doctor quickly looks for previous ECG results. Yes, the one from seven years ago is not showing any signs of an infarction! This news is ruffling the doctor's feathers. He decides to take immediate action—blood work and further tests of the heart. Geraldine is given center stage and describes in detail all the symptoms that have plagued her for the past week. The correct and highly targeted questions quickly point out that Geraldine might not be suffering from a common cold, but something much more sinister—a possible heart issue.

Based on the limited data from the ECG, it's close to impossible to say when the heart attack started. It might have happened three years ago, and Geraldine is now experiencing a nasty cold after all. Or it started seven days ago and is disguised as a nasty cold—impossible to say based on one ECG. The blood work will help us to be much more exact in our analysis. For now, Geraldine goes home while the doctor keeps an eagle eye on her blood results. After just a few hours, the doctor calls her to deliver the world-shattering diagnosis—a major myocardial infarction. For the past few days, blissfully unaware of the life-threatening illness, our tough grandma was brushing it off as a common cold!

The doctor takes all the necessary steps and immediately notifies the cardiologist on call. Geraldine packs her bags and, with her husband, heads straight to the ER. One intravenous drip later, the doctors are ready to proceed with an ultrasound examination of her heart. The bad news reverberates through the hospital room—Geraldine's heart function has drastically declined. Without wasting any time, she is wheeled into the operating theater, where doctors take an X-ray of her coronary arteries. The images show a series of quite drastic narrowings of the arteries. What now?

Working fast, the doctors use stents to immediately open the arteries and restore the blood flow. We are hoping for the best-case scenario: recovery! Unfortunately, Geraldine's condition is taking a turn for the worse. You see, the work on her coronary arteries has taken a toll on her already battered heart. Although the blood flow has been restored, the heart function is not showing any sign of improvement. Even the anesthesiologist needs to administer more and more supporting medications. Things are quickly taking a turn for the worse!

The doctors think on their feet and opt to implant an IABP (*intra-aortic balloon pump*), a short-term heart pump, to assist Geraldine's heart. They move mountains, and eventually it takes just three short minutes before the device is successfully implanted and switched on. In just fifteen minutes the supporting medication is already reduced, and Geraldine is transferred to the intensive care unit. She's alive, her coronary arteries are back open, and the IABP is helping her heart circulate oxygenated blood to her organs. Now we can exhale a sigh of relief and start examining her situation a bit closer.

The heart attack started a week ago. The blood flow through the coronary arteries has been restored, but the million-dollar question that lingers in the air is, "How much of Geraldine's heart muscle were we able to save?" Only time can tell us. Two weeks into her recovery, the results are in. The good news: the coronary arteries are still open, allowing ample blood flow. The bad news: Geraldine's heart muscle had suffered massive damage and still to this day is not showing any signs of recovery. As we are weaning the heart from the IABP's assistance, we quickly notice that it is slipping further away into the dangerous zone of terminal heart failure. Definitely bad news for the heart. What's the update on our patient's overall well-being?

You may be a bit surprised to hear this, but Geraldine is actually feeling quite well! She's radiating with happiness and is currently occupied with solving her favorite sudoku puzzles. It's quite self-explanatory that the big family reunion had to be rescheduled until further notice. Right now, Geraldine's husband is walking into her hospital room with a fresh pile of her favorite magazines. We are two weeks into her recovery, and we can already make a much better assessment. Geraldine is seventy-six years old and had absolutely no prior health conditions before she was stricken with her heart attack. As of today, pretty much all her organs have completely recovered—except her heart!

From the medical point of view, the best solution for Geraldine is to replace her IABP with an LVAD. The doctors just informed her about this option. From here on, the VAD (*ventricular assist device*) coordinator will guide her through it. VAD coordinators are highly trained specialists who guide and coach patients with long-term heart pumps. A heart specialist will work closely with a VAD coordinator in the same way an endocrinologist works with a dietician as they guide and advise a diabetic patient. Don't worry, later on we will put these people into much brighter spotlights and expand on their work in further detail.

Back to Geraldine, our VAD coordinator is doing his best to explain to Geraldine all the ins and outs of her LVAD. She needs to know everything: how the pump works, how many months and years it can function, what activities Geraldine can do and what she should definitely avoid—the list goes on. If you're curious about the full list, continue reading. We will take the time to learn all of it extensively later on.

Right now, Geraldine is absorbing all the new information that's fired at rapid succession. Remember, she's quite a tough and firm lady who's not intimidated by technology. She's a wonderful example to all senior citizens! Her unanimous decision is, "If this damn thing needs to be done, let's not waste time and get it over with!" Now the doctors can proceed. They remove the IABP and implant her new heart of steel that will take over the function of her left ventricle. The operation is a success! Just four weeks (and one pneumonia) later, Geraldine is finally heading home for the first time.

Geraldine's heart of steel is working flawlessly! Now she's ready to begin the long recovery that will take weeks. As you may imagine, implantation of such a complex device as an LVAD pump is quite a lengthy, complex, and heavy procedure that takes a toll on the patient's well-being. Now it's time for the long rehabilitation process, and we are 100 percent confident that Geraldine will be in top shape very soon. Since she doesn't fit the criteria for a heart transplantation, the heart of steel will be her permanent partner for many years to come. This is a perfect example of destination therapy (DT).

Scenario 5: Bridge to Recovery (BTR)

For us doctors, this scenario is the most fascinating and, unfortunately, the rarest of them all. We don't consider this scenario to be an active part of our strategy as we implant an LVAD. It's just something we really want to see as we follow up our patient's progress. What does this all mean?

You remember from previous chapters that heart failure progresses very gradually. When we see a case of end-stage heart failure, sometimes we can only stabilize it or slow it down using medication. A full recovery is usually impossible in this final stage. Or is it?

Sometimes, in very rare cases, we observe a peculiar phenomenon— patients with an LVAD start to show signs of complete reversal from their progressive heart failure. We call this *reverse remodeling*. If you remember from the previous chapters, remodeling occurs when the heart desperately tries to beef itself up in order to compensate for irreversible damage to the heart muscle. So in some patients we see the heart muscle getting leaner again, more cheetah than lion now, remember? If we happen to see the magical reverse remodeling in action, we can pop the cork and boldly proclaim that we are, in fact, dealing with a myocardial recovery!

The failing heart suddenly shows signs of self-regeneration—healing. In some rare cases, the heart can heal itself to the point of no longer needing the long-term heart pump at all. You read it correctly! Sometimes, in very rare cases, we can relieve the patient of their long-term heart pump entirely. Globally, this happens only in 1 percent of all cases. Although rare, this is a very well-known and well-documented phenomenon. Who are these lucky 1 percent?

Usually these are young people who are dealing with an inflammation of their heart muscle—myocarditis. When it comes to myocardial recovery of patients with a major myocardial infarction, let's just say that your chances of finding a gold nugget in your back garden are higher than seeing one of these people in person. These cases of the 1 percent are even more scarce! This incredible medical lottery is so unpredictable, it's almost impossible to know which patient has the chance of being a part of this lucky 1 percent. No matter what patient we're dealing with, we never lose hope and always look for signs of myocardial recovery. Every single time! What are those signs actually?

Just like a seasoned detective, we are looking for signs such as an increase in the contractility of the heart (an increase of the force of heart muscle contractions), the normalization of markers of heart failure in the blood samples, and the reshrinking of the expanded heart chambers (as the heart no longer needs to beef itself up to compensate for poor heart function due to heart muscle damage). Now imagine we find a lucky patient that ticks all the boxes. What now?

Yes, we can try to remove the LVAD as a part of the bridge to recovery scenario, but let's not get too far ahead of ourselves just yet. Let's keep in mind that this type of procedure is in fact a heavy operation. It will subject our patient to the risks of a redo surgery (with all the nasty adhesive tissue clinging on to the LVAD), not to mention the lengthy recovery process that inevitably follows. This is why we need to be confident that heart failure won't rear its ugly head later on in our patient's life. The choice we make together with our patient is literally a matter of life and death. We have to analyze both risks: life with an LVAD versus the potential redevelopment of heart failure later on in life. We will talk about these risks later on. Right now, it's time for the operation!

THE OPERATION

No matter what scenario our patients find themselves in, the procedure of implantation of an LVAD is always the same. The device is connected to the left ventricle, where it will suck blood, pressurize it, and direct the flow to the arteries. Right now, we'll roll up our sleeves and take a look at what a standard operation looks like. Then we will delve into the intricacies of several different variations of this operation. Ready?

Classic Implantation of an LVAD

First, the anesthesiologist will ensure our patient is in a deep artificial sleep. We'll ensure that there are several intravenous (IV) access points ready to administer the needed medication at a moment's notice. These IV access points also help if we need to proceed with an urgent blood transfusion. Next, we'll implant a special gauge to measure the blood flow. For now, this device will take up a temporary residence inside the pulmonary artery, where it will also measure the pulmonary pressures. Remember, the blood flow inside the pulmonary artery (coming from the right ventricle) is the same as inside the aorta (coming from the left ventricle). The right and left ventricles are two separate pumps that are connected in series. Let's move on.

Now we will proceed to slide an ultrasound probe into the patient's esophagus. This will allow us to have a look into the inside of the heart itself. Suddenly the inner workings of the atriums, ventricles, and valves become visible. Wonderful! Now let's disinfect our patient's skin. It goes without saying that in the field of heart surgery, we always work in sterile conditions. All of our equipment and surgical tools are thoroughly disinfected. LVADs, or any other artificial implant, for that matter, are quite beloved by bacteria. This is why we must go out of our way to avoid any and all potential infection vectors. Now we are ready to start our incisions.

We start with the middle of the chest. The skin in the center of the chest is cut from the small pit above the sternum to the bottom edge of that same sternum. Next we'll take a saw and cut through the sternum itself. Don't worry, it sounds a lot scarier than it actually is. After all, we need to gain access to the heart somehow, right?

Next, we will proceed to spread the sternum and create a cavity of 20 cm between both halves of the sternum. Now we have access to the mediastinum—the space between the sternum and both lungs. As you remember from Chapter 1, the heart is located inside the mediastinum, wrapped inside tissue that resembles a bag. This is the pericardium. As we open the pericardium, we finally gain access to the heart itself. You still remember that oxygen is life! Since we are going to implant the LVAD, we will need to temporarily ask the friendly heart-lung machine to take over all the heart and lung function of our patient. The heart-lung machine is actually a kind of ECMO machine but with a few adaptations specific to cardiac surgery. In cardiac surgery, the heart-lung machine is often referred to as the CPB (*cardio- pulmonary bypass*) because it allows the blood to bypass the patient's heart and lungs.

The CPB connection, in this case, will happen in the chest, close to the heart, not in the groin like an ECMO. Now we proceed to connect a tube of the CPB to the right atrium. The low-pressure blood from the venous system can now enter the CPB, receive ample oxygenation, and, after a quick pressurization, return to the patient's arteries and provide all the organs with enough oxygenated blood. This fresh blood enters directly into the patient's aorta via a second tube. Now the patient's bloodstream is connected to the CPB. We can let out a sigh of relief and start our evaluation of the heart itself.

The new long-term heart pump will live on the apex (the very tip of the heart) and will be connected directly to the left ventricle. We finally have ample time to analyze where and how this device will be implanted. Although we do have a bit of a wiggle room, we want to ensure the inflow cannula of the pump (the part that sucks the blood from the left ventricle) is precisely located in the middle of the left ventricle. Why? If this cannula is offset by just a tiny bit, it can suck the ventricular wall into it without any chance of releasing it. Imagine your vacuum cleaner sucking on a pillow and not letting it go. This is something we need to avoid at all costs. Let's find the golden spot, shall we?

Using our fingers, we'll push the tip of the heart inward. The anesthesiologist will see this physical motion transferred onto the screen—the area where our finger is pushing should be free from any obstructions! The golden spot is visible. Thank you, ultrasound probe in the esophagus! Time to use a special circular knife and remove a small area of the ventricular wall. This procedure is not for the squeamish! As the circular incision is made, we proceed to vacuum out the blood

Apical coring

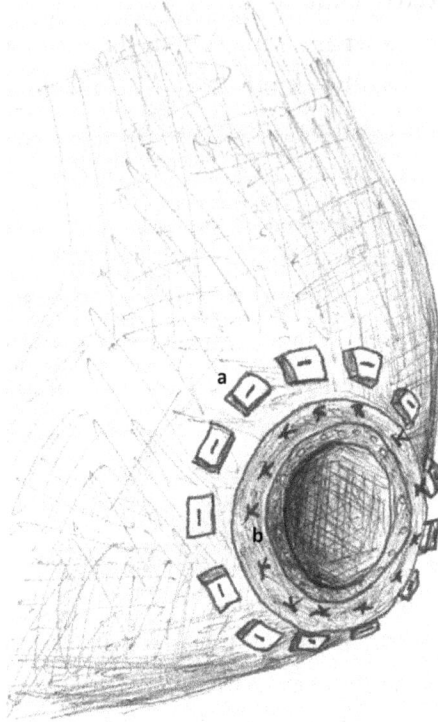

Figure 19.
With a special circular knife an incision is made at the apex of the left ventricle. With surgical sutures reinforced with Teflon pledgets (a), a metal ring (b) is connected to the opening. The LVAD will be clicked onto this metal ring.

from the left ventricle and inspect every part of the ventricle with an eagle eye. We're scouting for signs of blood clots. If we find any, we'll promptly remove them. Now, we can sew a special ring onto the circular incision we just made. This is where the entire pump unit will be clicked into place.

Now let's take care of the wiring. A heart pump runs on a continuous supply of electrical power. Currently, this power source lives outside of the patient's body. This is why we need to use the abdominal wall to guide this cable to the outside. First, we proceed with creating a pathway through the abdominal wall using a special probe. The cable starts at

Tunnel trajectory

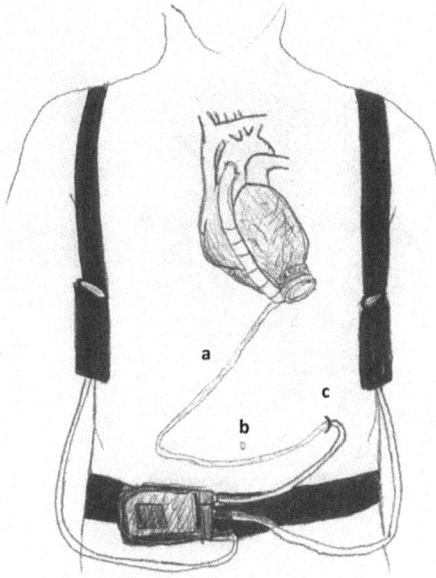

Figure 20.
The driveline starts at the LVAD attached to the heart. Its internal tunnel trajectory (a) starts behind the abdominal muscles. On the right side of the umbilicus (b) it reaches the subcutaneous tissues. It crosses over to the left side of the patient in the subcutaneus tissues under the umbilicus. At the left side of the umbilicus the cable exits the skin (c).

the upper end of the abdominal muscles (at the lower end of our chest incision). From there the cable follows a path to the right side of the belly button, circles back, and exits at the left side of the abdominal wall.

Why is this path so long and complicated? Short answer—protection against infections. Our skin barrier is a wonderful insulation against infections, protecting all of our internal tissues. The problems start when our cable reaches the outside world. From there bacteria start to creep up the cable toward the pump. The longer the trajectory between the outside world and the pump, the longer their journey takes and the more time we have to fight these bacteria. So, we can drastically reduce

LVAD connected to the heart

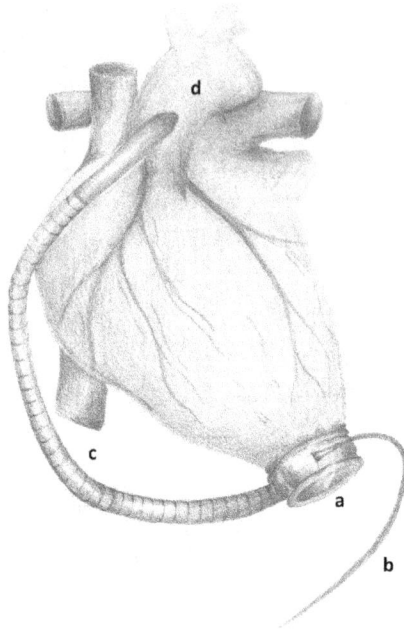

Figure 21.
The LVAD (a) is attached to the apex of the left ventricle. The device clicks onto a metal ring sewn to the apex. The driveline (b) will pierce the abdominal wall to connect to the controller. The outflow graft (c) is connected to the aorta (d).

the chance of infections making it to the heart itself. The cable is now in its correct position (nestled between our abdominal muscles and making some bends along the way to create more inner length). The cable is often referred to as the *driveline,* and the point where it exits the skin is called the *driveline exit site.*

Let's proceed to connect the heart pump itself. It needs to be connected to the arterial circulation of our patient's body. We make an incision in the aorta and sew the output tube of the heart pump to the aorta itself. This tube is called the *outflow graft,* and it will send pressurized blood directly to our patient's aorta and subsequently to all the needed organs.

Now our heart pump is fully connected with the heart and circulatory system of our patient. We are now ready to fire up the device.

This is quite a delicate process. We can't just rush it—it has to be done very gradually. Let's not forget that our CPB is still pumping blood through our patient's cardiovascular system! It's time to conduct a delicate mechanical orchestra where the CPB will stop its solo performance and fade into the background music while the long-term heart pump takes center stage. As we reduce the blood flow of the CPB, we increase this blood flow through our new steel heart. Suddenly an unexpected third violin enters the stage—the patient's heart itself!

You see, as we are decreasing the hard work of the CPB, the heart of the patient begins to beat as well. Now we are working with three blood pumps at the same time! There's no room for error at this stage. As the CPB stops entirely, we can proceed to disconnect the two tubes and allow the patient's heart to beat at a normal pace with the active assistance of the new steel heart. Suddenly things are a lot less complicated than before—now we can let our heart play with his new friend, the LVAD.

We can increase the speed of the steel heart using electrical signals (to allow more or less blood flow through), while the heart itself can be perfectly controlled using medication. It's time to tune both instruments to help find the best balance. This is the moment where the ultrasound probe in the esophagus and the measuring probe inside the pulmonary artery enter the center stage. From here it's their moment to shine and perform a crucial function in this operation. The images and values they provide will guide us through this process safely.

Once our tuning is completed, we finally achieve a stable situation. Now we can proceed to close up the pericardium and the sternum. As you may imagine, the heart and the heart pump are now one unit. The pericardium is simply too small to accommodate this new reality. This is why we use a special membrane made from an inorganic material to allow both pumps (heart and LVAD) ample room to coexist in perfect harmony. After this step is completed, we will use heavy steel wire to securely close our patient's sternum. As we are passing our second nerve-racking hour of the operation, we can finally wipe the sweat from our brow, exhale a sigh of relief, and send our patient to the intensive care (IC) unit. Success!

Currently our patient is still in a deep artificially induced sleep. In the IC unit, they will wake up very gradually. Sometimes the process of waking up can last hours. In some cases, even days! There are several factors at play that dictate these conditions, for example, how ill the patient was before their operation, how fit the patient's body is, and if there were any complications during the operation. We have to take into account every nitty-gritty detail. Again, there's no room for error. Now we can let our patient rest and wake up at their own pace.

From the moment our patient is finally awake and resumes a somewhat normal routine, they are ready to be transferred to a normal hospital room for rehabilitation and extensive education about all the intricacies of living with a heart pump. Maybe you are currently one of these people. Congratulations! You made it, and this is your second chance at life. Use it wisely. Live to your fullest extent and enjoy every moment your life has to offer. You won't regret it!

Perhaps you need a bit more time to recover, so why don't we take a moment to learn about alternative ways of implantation of the steel heart?

Alternative Implantations of the Heart Pump

In the world of surgical art, we always strive to make future procedures less heavy and invasive. This only brings further benefits to the patients. Today we have techniques such as keyhole surgeries and even robot-assisted surgery. These extremely high-tech sci-fi procedures are also present in heart surgery. It goes without saying that we can use these techniques in areas such as bypass surgeries and valve repair procedures. In these cases, we don't need to implant a large metallic object into the patient's chest cavity. The only thing going inside is a needle and some surgical wire. These tools will easily pass through the 1 centimeter keyholes.

A long-term heart pump is a completely different beast altogether. Those pesky laws of physics still don't allow us to implant a chunky piece of hardware using a 1 cm large incision. Luckily for patients from all over the world, medical science is constantly looking for new ways to reduce the size of the incisions during these implantation procedures. Smaller incisions mean less post-operative trauma for the patient. Less trauma means a speedy recovery and a happier patient. For example, there's a minimally invasive implantation whereby we'll approach the left ventricle through an incision between the ribs on the left side of the patient's chest. Through this smaller incision, we can eventually secure the pump to the left ventricle. What about the rest of the pump's plumbing?

The outflow graft can be sewn to the aorta using another less invasive method—by opening only the top side of the patient's sternum. No more need to open the entire chest. The recovery period can become progressively shorter, and this is, of course, music to any patient's ears! For now, it's fascinating to know that this method for heart pump implantation does exist. However, today it's not too popular. Some day in the future, perhaps this will change. As we perfect the new techniques, for now it's safe to say that we still cannot use the real keyhole surgery method for implantation procedures.

Many colleagues fail to see any benefits to this surgical innovation using smaller incision. I can definitely follow their reasoning. Contrary to popular belief, a sternotomy (the process of opening the sternum to gain access to the patient's heart) is not as invasive as many people think. You see, most patients recover extremely well, without signs of pain or discomfort. Sadly, the same can't be said about an incision between the ribs. This actually tends to be more painful for the patient during their rehabilitation.

Another benefit of a full-on sternotomy is easier access to the aorta—we have ample space to work and control potential bleeding events should they occur during surgery. In the end, it's up to the surgeon himself to decide the best and safest option for the patient. The bottom line is, both classic surgery and the less invasive type have the same long-term results: a second chance at life for our patients.

Additional Procedures During LVAD Implantation

When patients have had cardiac surgery, they sometimes brag about how big the surgery was: "I had five bypasses!" or "They had to work on three valves." So can we give our heart pump patients some extra tools for bragging, or is an LVAD implantation a solitary procedure? In most cases it is "just" the implantation of the LVAD, but in some patients we need to do a little extra.

Valve Surgery

Some patients will have heart valves that are not working properly. Most common in heart failure patients, we see a leaking mitral valve (the valve between the left atrium and left ventricle). In chronic heart failure, the left ventricle is dilated, and this stretches the mitral valve, causing an improper closing of the valve and leakage of blood to the left atrium. So do we need to repair this valve? Some people do, but in most cases this leakage disappears naturally after the heart pump is implanted. Two mechanisms contribute to this. First, the inflow cannula sucks the blood away from the mitral valve, greatly reducing the backflow over this valve. Second, the LVAD unloads the failing left ventricle and reduces the dilatation. This in turn relieves the stretch of the mitral valve, improving its function.

Another valve that might leak is the tricuspid valve (the valve between the right atrium and right ventricle). Need a reminder about the valves? Scroll back to Figure 3 in the first chapter for an overview! We often see the degree of leakage of the tricuspid valve diminishing after an LVAD implantation because the right ventricle has an easier time pumping blood over the lungs (the lung resistance decreases with the implantation of a heart pump on the left side). But the effect is smaller than in the mitral valve. So if we have a DT patient with severe tricuspid regurgitation, we might opt to repair this valve.

Another valve that might cause problems is the aortic valve. The aortic valve sits neatly between our left ventricle and the aorta. As you remember, this important part of our anatomy prevents pressurized blood from flowing back into the left ventricle during diastole (as the heart muscle relaxes and prepares for the next pump). Thanks to this important valve, the blood is always flowing in one direction, from the ventricle to the aorta.

Aortic valve insufficiency occurs as the leaflets of the aortic valve don't close properly. The result of this is blood flowing back into the left ventricle. In general, healthy people can handle a light degree of aortic valve insufficiency. However, when it comes to patients with a steel heart, this condition cannot be ignored. If left untreated, potential complications are destined to come knocking on the front door after some time. Let's take a moment to dive a bit deeper into this important condition.

As this valve is malfunctioning, there will be some flowback of blood from the aorta into the left ventricle. If we follow the blood flow, we can observe that it flows from the left ventricle through the LVAD into the aorta and subsequently (due to the leaky aortic valve) back into the left ventricle. So, in essence, the leaky aortic valve is creating a small, closed loop of blood flow. As you may imagine, our body doesn't benefit from this looping blood flow at all. On the contrary—the efficiency of the LVAD reduces significantly. But that's not even the least of our problems. What happens next?

As the leaky aortic valve allows some blood to return to the left ventricle, this important chamber becomes filled up to the max. Nothing can be stretched to its limit without consequences, so naturally, with time, the mitral valve can start showing signs of leaking as well. After all, the left ventricle has to do something with all this extra blood, right? As the mitral valve starts to leak, more blood will start to flow back into the pulmonary circulation, wreaking havoc on our lungs. Before you know it, the good old friend pulmonary edema is knocking on the door with some worrying consequences—fluid buildup inside our lungs.

As you now clearly understand, this dangerous chain reaction is something we need to avoid at all costs, especially inside the body of a patient with a steel heart. The natural question that arises is, "What can we do to avoid aortic valve insufficiency?" Imagine that we already know that the aortic valve is showing signs of weakness even before we start our surgery. Especially in the somewhat older patients, we can see calcified valves that don't open and close that well anymore. In this case, we will address this issue by replacing the valve with a *biological artificial valve.*

Again, don't be intimidated by the medical terminology. *Biological* simply means that the valve is made from bovine pericardial tissue. It's an ideal material to work with because it's so similar to our native aortic valve. Great news! Now we finally solved the issue, right? Well, things are not that simple.

The good news is that we can expect our patient to live a carefree ten to fifteen years with their biological aortic valve. The bad news is that we are working with biological material that is susceptible to aging and subsequent malfunctioning after that period of time. Surely there should be other options out there? Maybe something that can last for thirty to forty (maybe even fifty) years?

Yes, there are mechanical valves out there. But before you consider going full-on cyborg, you should hear about the drawbacks of this solution. Every time a mechanical valve closes, it will emit a distinctive ticking sound. Try closing your water tap rapidly, and you will hear something similar. In 90 percent of the cases, patients don't hear this sound, but for the other 10 percent, this becomes a living hell. You hear ticking every second, every hour, or every day—enough to put Edgar Allan Poe's *The Tell-Tale Heart* to shame. Not fun and not something we would want our patients to go through.

Another drawback of the mechanical valves is the need for quite strong blood thinners, the vitamin K antagonists, which we will talk about later. When we opt for a biological artificial valve, you won't need any stronger blood thinning medications than those needed for your LVAD.

A last point in favor of the biological valves is that when the valve eventually begins to fail, it can now be replaced by an endovascular valve.

Some of our patients exhibit a peculiar phenomenon—the valve leaflets are perfectly fine, yet the valve itself does not properly close.

Park stitch

Before

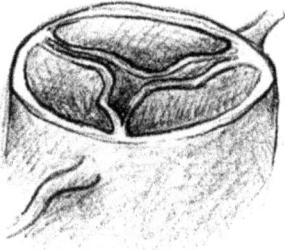

After

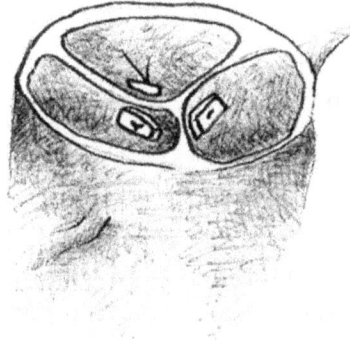

Figure 22.
When the aortic valve is insufficient due to the lack of central coaptation of the valve leaflets, this can be addressed with the Park stitch. The central portion of the three leaflets are tied together with a stitch. This closes the central portion of the valve and erases the insufficiency.

Often this malcoaptation finds itself in the very center of the valve (creating leakage and backflow). In the case that this leaking is minimal and doesn't hinder the young patient, we won't risk any additional surgical procedure. "Just" an LVAD implantation only and allow our patient to wait for a replacement heart on the transplant waiting list.

Sometimes, though, the situation is quite different. Imagine that our patient is a DT (destination therapy) candidate or suffering from a more severe valve backflow. In this case we'll sew the valve leaflets together in the center. This technique is called the Park stitch (named after the doctor who developed it). In summary, by stitching the three valve leaflets in the center, we will prevent the leaking and blood backflow entirely. In the case that our DT patient still has any heart function left, the valve will still allow for blood flow to pass freely through the open sides of the valve leaflets.

In some special cases we can even opt to close the aortic valve entirely. As you remember, this is perfectly possible because our LVAD is sending blood from the left ventricle directly to our aorta (bypassing the aortic valve). This method is used on patients with a prior history of serious aortic valve surgeries. From a technical point of view, it's a lot safer to close off the valve using a special type of surgical patch rather than performing complex additional surgery on a valve you can miss as an LVAD patient.

Atrial Septal Defect

In the womb, all of us have a hole in the interatrial septum (the wall between the right and the left atrium). Soon after birth, this closes naturally in most people, but sometimes a little defect remains. Nothing to worry about. I'm sure many readers of this book have it without even knowing it, and it will probably never cause them any harm. But in heart pump patients, it sometimes needs to be addressed. Why? The pressure in the left atrium is higher compared to the right atrium, meaning that if blood is flowing over the atrial septal defect, it will flow from left to right. Blood from the left atrium has just passed the lungs and is rich in oxygen. Now as we implant an LVAD and turn up the pump speed, it reduces the pressure in the left atrium, sometimes even lower than the pressure in the right atrium. According to the laws of physics, flow is driven by the pressure difference, so the flow might now even reverse, from the right atrium to the left atrium. This blood from the right atrium just delivered all of its oxygen to our body and is thirsty for a top-up with fresh oxygen in the lungs. But as it is sucked down the atrial septal defect, this will not happen. For our patient, this means that the blood that is pumped from the left ventricle to the systemic circulation is carrying less oxygen, and oxygen is life! So let's close this defect as we find it!

HEART PUMPS FOR THE SMALLEST PATIENTS

Contrary to popular belief, not only adults are under attack from heart failure. Unfortunately, this condition can occur in children as well—sometimes even at quite an early age. Within cardiac surgery, children are an entirely separate discipline. Their heart defects are oftentimes structural in nature. In other words, the anatomy of a child's sick heart is often different. Naturally, we need quite different surgical techniques to help these small patients to the best of our ability. But strangely enough, it is often not those anatomically different hearts that fail at a young age.

We have seen how the doctors solved Lucas's heart defect at a very young age. As our patient grows up, a young heart (even while the right ventricle is doing all the heavy lifting and supporting the systemic circulation) can handle this strange new reality. However, after a certain time, because even the best and healthiest heart can only take so many hard punches, it slowly descends into heart failure. By this time, the babies have already long grown up into fully functional adults.

Today, most of our young patients who qualify for the steel heart are either suffering from genetic heart defects (that don't allow the heart muscle to function properly) or from myocarditis (inflammation of the heart muscle). If we examine these tiny hearts from a strictly medical point of view, we can safely conclude that they are structurally (meaning anatomically) normal. In theory, this should make the implantation procedure of an LVAD perfectly possible. Again, only in theory! You see, the heart of a child is significantly smaller than that of a full-grown adult. If operating on an eight-year-old patient can be considered challenging, and for babies weighing just 3 kg (6.61 lbs.), this procedure is simply impossible. It goes without saying that we can't just ignore the needs of these tiny patients. Instead, we will opt for an external heart pump that will keep our patients alive and in good health. This allows us ample time to work out a strategy that will fit the needs of the child as they grow up and mature. Depending on the age, these are solutions that fit the needs of every patient. Let's see how it all works.

Babies, Toddlers, and Preschoolers
To say that operating on such fragile patients is challenging is a massive understatement. As you may imagine, the thorax of our smallest

patients is just a tiny bit larger than the size of an adult steel heart device. Luckily, we have external heart pumps that are perfectly suited to save the little rascals. This specialized artificial heart pump lives fully outside of the child's body with only four tubes that connect the heart to the device. Two tubes are connected to the atriums or ventricles (surgeon's preference) of the right and left heart and deliver blood to the pump.

We use a classic pulsatile pump with one-way valves (that you already know from the previous chapters or have a look at Figure 17 again). Although a bit old school, it works well, and it allows us to mimic a somewhat natural heartbeat. The blood enters a hollow chamber that's divided by a membrane. On the other side of the membrane, gas is rhythmically pushing (and releasing), creating a pumping action. Just like a classic bellows, these pumps have been around for a long time. As the pump is fired up, and we can follow the blood flow.

As the blood is pressurized by the pump, it follows along two tubes toward the pulmonary artery (the large artery that feeds our lungs) and to the aorta. As you already may have guessed, this is how we support the two main blood circulatory systems of our tiny patient—the pulmonary and systemic circulation. If we want to be perfectly correct, we should mention the putative pump is composed of two separate pumps—each responsible for the designated circulatory system. For the sake of full transparency, it's important to mention that these pumps are not completely free from risks. Due to their design, there are risks of blood clots inside the pump body and on the one-way valves.

Speaking of risks, let's not forget that we are working with four exposed tubes (all of them thicker than the driveline of a modern implantable heart pump) that all exit the body of our small patient. This alone is a massive risk for infection! Luckily, this is merely a temporary solution. You see, the children who are unfortunate enough to need the assistance of this heart pump are very quickly put on the waiting list for an urgent heart transplantation.

When it comes to adults, it's safe to say that we can conduct an urgent heart transplantation within two weeks (in Belgium). When it comes to small children, this is an entirely different story. There are simply not many donors out there; hence the waiting lists can be longer. In Belgium these patients usually receive a donor heart within months.

During this waiting period, the small baby will have to remain in the intensive care unit at the hospital, chained to the artificial heart that rhythmically pumps the blood through the tiny body. Luckily, as the babies grow up, they will probably not have any conscious memories of this quite invasive experience. Ask any person if they would like the idea of remembering such an event. The answer would be a firm and unanimous, "No!"

At this very moment, some companies are developing small LVADs suitable for children. It's important to keep in mind that these devices are still somewhat too large for our smallest patients, yet for larger children, they can mean all the difference in the world. Having a small *and* implantable LVAD opens the doors to the much-needed mobility that all children crave as they set out exploring the world around them. We are holding on to our hearts (pun intended) to see new and exciting developments for babies, toddlers, and preschoolers.

Children

They grow up so fast, don't they? Any parent knows it all too well, and this is why we truly cherish every moment together. As a preschooler grows into a child, we can start to consider the use of a fully adult size steel pump from the age of eight or nine years old. Strictly from the medical point of view, it's quite important to properly prepare for every scenario. Sometimes it can be tricky to obtain ample space inside the chest of our patient. This is why we take the necessary time scanning and gauging every part of the thorax just to have a better understanding of what is physically possible to achieve with a surgical procedure. We take no chances and will only proceed when we are sure that the implantation has a high chance of success.

Remember that the heart remodels itself during the long period of progressive heart failure? This beefed up and enlarged heart is much larger than a healthy one, and it already takes up a significant amount of space at the expense of the internal organs inside the chest. Naturally, as we implant the steel heart and allow it to assist the left ventricle of the failing heart, the pump will suck blood out of the enlarged ventricle, and it will start to shrink to a more normal size. So more room for the LVAD! For surgeons and our tiny patients, this is music to our ears!

You may ask yourself if children are expected to live for many years with their steel hearts assisting their left ventricles. The short answer is no! We will only use the implantation surgery as a bridge to transplantation scenario. The sooner we find a donor heart for our child patient, the better. Let's meet one of them, shall we?

Noah is a ten-year-old rascal. He's a talented basketball player and happens to be training at one of the best basketball clubs Belgium has to offer. The past couple of weeks Noah's coach noticed something peculiar—the kid is lacking his usual oomph during training. In the past Noah was number one—lightning fast and agile, today he's in last place. What the hell is happening? Noah decides to talk to his parents. Luckily for him, they have also noticed their son's lack of luster. He's been lingering in his room, and something just felt off. It's time to visit the family physician.

The doctor notices Noah's elevated heartbeat but can't put his finger on what's causing all the discomfort and loss of energy and youthful vibe. As a family physician, he's intimately acquainted with Noah's family. He knows that the kid is passionate about becoming a top-performing athlete. The doctor concludes that he must have just pushed himself too hard. The kid should focus more on school and spend less time shooting hoops with his friends. The doctor recommends skipping two weeks of practice, allowing Noah to rest and recover.

Noah's parents and the family physician may still be lingering in a haze of blissful ignorance, but you already suspect that something much more sinister is lurking in the shadows. You're right—Noah is suffering from cardiomyopathy! Fast-forward one week, and Noah's condition is quickly deteriorating. Aside from a loss of appetite, he's also suffering from shortness of breath as a high fever rages through his body. His parents sound the alarm and deliver their son to the emergency room.

What would you think if you were an emergency doctor who saw a ten-year-old child who was coughing and violently shivering with a high fever? Probably pneumonia, right? The doctor orders a chest x-ray and blood work while he prepares the list of necessary antibiotics. Currently he's not doubting his diagnosis. Yes, the kid is in pretty bad shape, but that doesn't mean he will need to be admitted. Just one hour later, as the emergency doctor checks the test results, he's finally confronted with the severity of the situation. Now it's the doctor's turn to shiver!

Noah's lungs are filled with fluid, and his heart has grown to twice the size of a normal heart! It's safe to say that this is not normal pneumonia. This is much more serious! The doctor calls a colleague cardiologist who (at last) correctly diagnoses Noah's condition as heart failure! The heart function is drastically reduced, and as an overcompensation mechanism, the heart has beefed itself up, making it too large. This looks like a case of myocarditis (inflammation of the heart muscle) or a genetic defect that has been showing its presence after years of slumber. Finding the cause of Noah's heart failure becomes a second priority. Right now, the kid needs urgent help! Off to the intensive care unit . . .

First, Noah is connected to intravenous medication drips—this medication will support his heart and hopefully bring him some much-needed relief. Sadly, his heart failure has progressed past the stage where any medication will help to alleviate any symptoms. The next day a team of heart surgeons, pediatricians, cardiologists, and anesthetists bow their heads over Noah's condition.

Yes, the young patient is suffering from a serious, life-threatening condition. All the treatment options available are drastic, invasive, and not always risk-free. Contrary to popular belief, there isn't any single rock star doctor who can correctly decide the best treatment. Only a team of qualified specialists is capable of gauging all available methods at their disposal. As of now, medication is off the table. The second option is a catheter-mounted heart pump. Let's quickly explore this option.

If you remember Peter, this was his best solution, but goddamn it, he was a fully mature twenty-year-old man at the time of the operation.

We're dealing with a ten-year-old child. Noah's great blood vessels are simply too small to use as a delivery system for even the smallest heart pump we have at our disposal. What now? The IABP and ECMO are still left unexplored. If you remember the previous chapters, you'll already know that an IABP just simply won't cut it. It won't be able to offer Noah's heart ample assistance to increase his chances of recovery. IABP is off the table. What about ECMO?

Yes, we can connect the large, bulky machine to his blood circulatory system, but that comes at a cost. Will an active ten-year-old boy be able to remain chained to a bed for ten days? He will, but only while being submerged in an artificial coma. Another side effect of the ECMO is that it will work against Noah's heart. This means we're looking at risks of having lazy blood in the left ventricle. Definitely not a good option! Our favorite solution (catheter-mounted heart pump) cannot even fit through the young patient's narrow arteries. Every possibility for short-term pumps has been depleted. Let's move on, no time to waste!

Option 5 (after medications, catheter-mounted pumps, IABP and ECMO have been ruled out)—waiting list for a heart transplantation. Sadly, time is a luxury we don't have. We need a solution today, and every hour that passes, Noah's life is hanging by a thread. What is the chance that a donor heart will magically appear right here, right now? The boy's body has been putting up such a brave fight against heart failure that it has completely depleted itself. Subjecting Noah to a heart transplant surgery is simply too damn risky. What else is out there?

Enter option 6—the LVAD implantation. This procedure can be performed immediately. If we choose to proceed, we can even acquire a tissue sample of Noah's heart muscle while we are performing the operation. We can send that piece of tissue over to the pathologist. This will increase our chances of finding the cause of Noah's heart failure later on. With a laser-focused diagnosis, Noah may even get the chance to make it into the BTR (bridge to recovery) scenario where a donor heart would not be needed in the first place. Let's hope for the best!

Right now, we need to hurry. The medical team has weighed the risks and benefits of all options and unanimously agreed to proceed with option 6. Now that the starter pistol shot has been fired, it sets in motion a medical sprint to save the life of our young protagonist. Everything is prepared for Noah's arrival into the operating theater . . .

Fast-forward four months, and the beads of nervous sweat are already visible on the forehead of the VAD coordinator as he exhales a heavy sigh. Yes, today Noah comes to bless him with his presence—during another scheduled consultation. This kid can give a Labrador puppy a run for his money! He can't sit still for a single second. The untapped curiosity and wonder send the happy child on a quest to discover every corner of the doctor's office. He asks questions about all the "cool gear" that the VAD coordinator happens to have lying around. He wants to push all the buttons and try out all the tech. In short, a few more gray hairs for the VAD coordinator and a hell of a lot of good news for Noah!

The LVAD steel heart has saved the kid's life, and now he's back to his old jolly self—overflowing with energy and youthful optimism. Today his name will appear on the heart transplant waiting list. Just eight months later he has a fully functional donor heart. Although being a basketball star will probably be a bit out of reach for Noah, we can't deny the obvious—the LVAD saved his life! Now he can fully embrace the future and take his life by the horns.

CHAPTER 6

LIVING WITH A HEART PUMP

A PATIENT THAT JUST RECEIVED THEIR LVAD IMPLANT can honestly be considered luckier than any lottery winner in the world. Think about it! In essence, you just cheated death and can now enjoy your second life (that until now perhaps you took for granted). A heart pump is an incredibly sophisticated electro-mechanical orchestra of parts all working together in perfect harmony with only one mission— keeping you alive!

Your LVAD will require effort and discipline from your side. If you neglect it, you *will* die! During the first months, some patients can experience a somewhat awkward adjustment period. However, after a while it all becomes second nature, just like breathing. In this chapter we will take a closer look at all the intricacies of living with your new heart pump. We'll break down every strange ritual and custom that will very soon become just a normal part of your daily routine.

THE PUMP

The mechanical pump itself doesn't have an onboard battery or any computer built into its housing. Remember the long trajectory of the cable that runs through the abdominal wall? As this cable exits the patient's abdomen, it is connected to a small external device. This is the control unit of your LVAD. It is connected to two separate batteries.

As you may have guessed, this connection between the cable and the controller is permanent. If this connection is severed, the pump stops working!

The cable is quite tough and reinforced to handle the physical stresses of daily life. In the case of a potentially severed connection, there will be a loud audible alarm that the patient cannot miss or ignore. Let's move on to the controller. This is a small box that houses an entire computer designed to provide your heart pump with a fixed speed and power. This computer monitors the pump's performance at all times. If some parameters are off from normal, you will again be reminded of this with a loud alarm tone. The controller will meticulously record the event so the data can be analyzed later on during a hospital visit.

As you see, there are several fail-safes and alarms built into this amazing machine. One of the most important alarms is called a *suction alarm*. This is triggered when the pump excerpts too much vacuum force on the inside of the ventricle—effectively sucking the ventricle shut. In these rare cases, the controller will detect it, and the pump will automatically decrease its speed for a short period of time. This results in less suction force after a couple of seconds. Now the left ventricular wall can come free from the inflow cannula. Problem solved, and both the heart and the pump will resume their normal function.

Just like with all electrical devices, batteries run lower and lower during normal operation. A phone shutting down due to an empty battery might seem the end of the world to an influencer, but an empty battery in an LVAD really can end your time in this world. No wonder low battery status triggers an alarm. Another important alarm will sound when the blood flow of the heart pump drops below 2.5L per minute or when the controller detects something fishy that deviates from normal operation of the pump. All these sorts of abnormalities are too important to ignore, which is why we spend so much time educating patients and their partners on how to handle these situations correctly. We will do our best to explain every type of alarm, the severity of the situation, and of course how to handle it during daily life.

LVAD peripherals

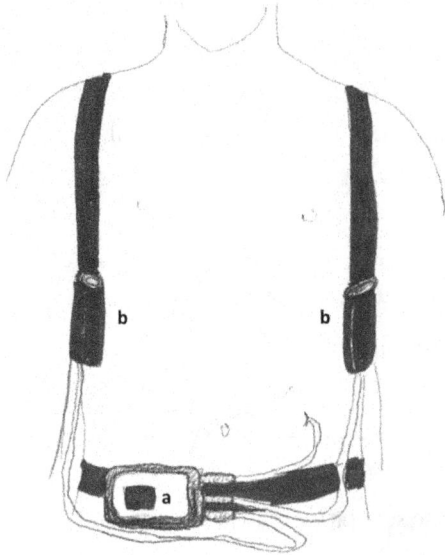

Figure 23.
The LVAD is connected to the controller by the driveline. The controller (a) has two cables connected to two external battery packs (b) providing power to the LVAD

For example, there are orange and red alarms. The red one is, of course, much more serious than the orange one! At any time during such an alarm, you can take a glimpse at the controller and gauge the situation. The controller will always show the status of the pump: if it is still pumping blood, the overall status of the unit, and much more.

The controller also provides power to the heart pump. A patient with a long-term heart pump will have several options for providing power to their heart pump. There are batteries, wall outlets, and even car battery adapters. Whatever situation life throws at you, your heart pump will be able to work perfectly. When it comes to going mobile and using just the batteries, at any given time you will have a respectable twelve to sixteen hours of uninterrupted mobility. Out of precaution, we always recommend that patients carry at least one set of spare batteries with them at all times. You never know when it may come in handy!

As you walk the streets with your heart pump, you'll always be carrying some hardware with you. Both batteries have a combined weight of just 1.2 kg and take no more space than a lunch box. Let's not forget our control unit. In total there will be three packs. In the past patients relied on heavy nickel-cadmium batteries, while today the lighter lithium-ion batteries ensure much greater mobility.

Let's see the total weight of your heart pump setup:

- The control unit is just under 500 grams.
- The two batteries are around 600 grams each.
- The pump with driveline and graft is a small 300 grams.

That equals out to around 2 kg of additional weight you have to carry with you.

In the past these setups were quite bulky, but thanks to the technological advancements in medical science, we were able to shed plenty of weight from the overall system. This is definitely amazing news for the patients. Now, how do we go about carrying these essential items?

Some patients prefer to keep their controllers and batteries hidden away in special pouches that live on their belts. Other people prefer to use a shoulder bag. Some creative minds even convert their backpacks and purses to accommodate their heart pump hardware. Whatever a patient feels comfortable with is the right choice.

When it comes to modification of accessories, we need to keep in mind that the controller *always* remains securely connected to the cable that exits the patient's abdomen. This cable is a bit longer than 40 cm (15.74"). Yes, there's a bit of wiggle room, but it doesn't mean that a patient can simply drop all the gear in a backpack and swing it across their shoulder. There are some intricacies that need some special attention.

For example, it's always a good idea to modify the clothing to allow the cable (and the control unit) to pass seamlessly to the outside. This way it can be slipped into a pouch or a carry case of your choice. It's quite self-explanatory that some patients may struggle with the battle between comfortable clothing and the practicality of carrying their control unit and batteries. For people who love dresses, this can definitely be a challenge—you will need a certain degree of modification of your garments.

One of our patients is a seamstress. Today she's giving helpful advice to fellow patients on how to overcome these challenges. Some patients chose to do away with all these modifications and simply chose to wear special underwear or shirts to suit their needs. These garments are specially outfitted with pockets that allow for safe and convenient storage for both the control unit and batteries.

And just like magic, there's no more fidgeting around with garments trying to feed the control unit through the dress or jacket, no more need for bags, backpacks, and purses. From the outside, nobody would even suspect that you're walking around packing all that hardware for your heart pump. You may already guess that young people usually prefer this solution above all else. Before you rejoice at the prospect of never needing bags and backpacks, Steve Jobs would say, "There's one more thing!" If you are walking around with an undergarment that houses your heart pump's necessities and you hear an audible alarm, this means you'll need to find a private space to undress and inspect your control unit.

As you finish your day and head back home, there's an option to use an external wall socket as a power source. The length of this adapter cable is 6 m (20 feet), and it's connected to the charging station for your batteries. This may seem like a lot but try to manage your household on a 20-foot leash, and you'll be surprised how short that actually is! The best way to use the wall outlet is to use it while you sleep. This allows patients to experience the least amount of discomfort and get a good night's sleep. Again, if your nightly rest is interrupted by the call of nature, this means some fidgeting is required to unplug your wall outlet cable and take your battery with you.

By now you hopefully understand that for many patients, their

LVADs are literally their best friends, as well as their mortal enemies. Daily life with an LVAD requires some attention, and behavior needs to be modified to suit the inconveniences of this amazing tech. Just like that voice of reason that lives in your head, the heart pump is with you 24/7, literally keeping you alive! In the beginning, many patients panic at the sound of the alarm, yet with time they learn to live with their heart pump and accept the new routine in the same way you would brush your teeth in the morning and not even think about it.

One thing is certain: a patient living with a heart pump values every moment of every day. When you look past all the inconveniences and behavioral modifications, you understand that you are alive and well. Just a few short decades ago, this was science fiction. Now, it is a perfectly normal reality for thousands of people around the world.

THE FOLLOW-UP PROCESS

When our patient is implanted with a shiny new LVAD, after a certain time they will head home to start their second life. It goes without saying that the hospital staff will be ever so vigilant and schedule their follow-up meetings. There's a small army of specialized nurses and VAD coordinators that direct the daily orchestra of following the patient's progress. This happens inside the hospital walls as well as out in the wild. All these specialists share a round table together with the patient's physicians and help to guide every case to a successful outcome.

What about the VAD coordinators? They are specialized in educating the patients on all the intricacies of their shiny new steel hearts. For example, they teach the patient the importance of wound care—the driveline that exits the patient's abdomen needs to be squeaky clean at all times. They explain the inner workings of the control unit, and they coach the patient on the use of the correct medications.

As if this wasn't enough, a VAD coordinator will even accompany the patient to their home. Inside the walls of the patient's dwelling, they will help to install all the supporting hardware for the heart pump and inform the patient's family physician and the nurse who will be visiting the patient on a regular basis. Many family physicians are not fully aware of all the intricacies of LVADs. We're dealing with quite sophisticated and still "new" technology—the more information we give to patients and doctors, the better! I sincerely hope this book will also help you in this regard. Let's head back to the patient's home.

Here, the patient will have two important responsibilities—wound care (of the driveline exit site) and blood-thinning medications. If you remember the chapter about blood, you'll know that we want to avoid blood clots in the pump at all times. This is where blood thinners come in. The ones traditionally used in patients with a heart pump are the so-called *vitamin K antagonists*—they block vitamin K production inside the liver. This vitamin K is needed to produce blood-clotting factors. No vitamin K—no risk of blood clots! Done deal, right? Not quite . . .

You see, this type of blood thinner has a very important drawback: not every patient will experience the same effect from the same dose of medication. For example, a single 5 mg tablet a day would be too much for one patient and too little for another. To make things worse, the requirements can also change over time in a single patient. So whatever was the right dose six months ago might now be too much or too little. This peculiar problem is solved by carefully measuring the blood clotting factors of every patient and modifying our medication doses accordingly. In the past, it was quite a cumbersome process—once or even twice a week the patient had to visit their family physician to draw some blood and run the needed tests. Today, you can do it at home with just a tiny drop of blood drawn from your finger, just like a diabetes patient measures the sugar levels in their blood.

Thanks to miracles of technology, all the current patients who are living with heart pumps can determine the right dosage of needed medication from the comfort of their homes and even input all the values into a special app. We have to thank our hospital for developing this proprietary app! It tells the patient the exact number of tablets that need to be taken based on the measurements from a simple finger prick. The app also instructs the patient when the next scheduled blood measurement is taking place.

In some rare cases we have to stop administering blood thinners altogether. This happens, for example, when a patient needs to undergo a surgical procedure. Performing surgery whilst the patient is on vitamin K antagonists brings a high risk of bleeding during the surgery. In this case, the tablets are replaced with another type of blood thinner that has a shorter working time. This type of blood thinner has to be injected into subcutaneous tissue. By timing the injections correctly, we can perform surgery with a low risk of bleeding and, at the same time, minimize the risk of blood clots forming in the LVAD.

As you already know, medical science never sleeps! Recently, new types of blood thinners became available for patients with a heart pump. A patient can now profit from something called a NOAC. Again, don't let the confusing terminology throw you off guard. NOAC simply stands for *non-vitamin K oral anticoagulants*. Let's eat this elephant one bite at a time!

This medication is designed in a way that doesn't block the production of vitamin K inside the liver. Hence the name non-vitamin K oral anticoagulants. Suddenly one (or two tablets) per day is enough to achieve the same effect—prevention of blood clots. And the best part is, no more finger prick required! We only have to determine the right dose once you start taking this NOAC. Thereafter, you can just continue that dose for life. This is definitely good news. What's the bad news then? Unfortunately, this new medication is not as powerful as the classic one. For a long time, doctors thought that a NOAC wasn't powerful enough to prevent blood clotting from occurring inside the heart pump. When we're dealing with older designs of heart pumps, this is absolutely true.

Today, things have changed for the better. Thanks to new designs of the heart pumps, an NOAC is more than sufficient for the job—this is music to the ears of our patients! A little side note to be complete, NOACs are now often referred to as DOACs (*direct oral anticoagulants*). Different name but exactly the same drug!

Now you know about the medication, let's take a look at the driveline that powers the LVAD. As you know, this driveline exits the patient's abdomen. We took great care to make the path of this cable as long as possible on the inside of our patient's abdomen. The long trajectory of the cable is the second-best protection against possible infections. The first method of protection is, of course, the patient himself. As the cable exits the abdominal wall, the integrity of the skin is suddenly breached. This driveline exit site is a potential hazard for bacterial infection, and we need to address it accordingly. Why exactly?

When bacteria linger on the cable's surface and settle in their new habitat, they might get too comfortable and start to replicate. A few bacteria can be handled by our immune system, but massive numbers are a different story, and they can cause a serious infection. These types of infections are an absolute nightmare to treat, so we'll follow the age-old practice that states, "Prevention is better than a cure." Naturally, this means we will spend ample time nursing the area where the cable exits the patient's abdominal wall. It needs all the care and attention in the world. We will educate the patient on how to handle this delicate task properly. If the patient can't handle this important task on their own, we'll call in the "flying angels" (home nurses) to help. It's important not to understate the seriousness of a potential infection! Consider this, if an infection does occur, we will need to treat it with proper antibiotics. In the worst case, a patient will have to rely on the use of these antibiotics for a very long time—sometimes even for life! Again, prevention is much better than a cure!

Every patient is different, and every case we handle can be considered unique in some respects. When it comes to medications, aside from the normal blood thinners, there are some other important medications that we cannot ignore when dealing with patients suffering from heart failure. One of the most important ones are medications that regulate blood pressure. As you now know, when the heart pump is happily buzzing away, the pulse pressure (the difference between systolic and diastolic pressure) will drastically reduce—sometimes even to 0. In essence, we don't feel the patient's pulse, while there clearly is pressure present inside the circulatory system. This is where highly sensitive blood pressure monitors come in. These machines can accurately read all the patient's values in real time.

You may remember how we measure blood pressure—using the column of mercury method. In ideal situations we aim to keep the blood pressure lower than 100 mmHg. This is quite low compared to the blood pressure of people who live without a long-term heart pump. Their normal systolic blood pressure is usually 120 mmHg. When the values jump to 140 mmHg (or higher), we can consider this already too high. These numbers change drastically when we're looking at patients with a long-term heart pump.

For example, the normal blood pressure in a patient with a heart pump is between 80 and 90 mmHg. After extensive studies, our medical colleagues have discovered that anything over 100 mmHg results in a higher risk of strokes. Conclusion: when you live with a long-term heart pump, it's definitely a good idea to keep an eye on the correct blood pressure.

What about the heart pump itself? A higher pressure is also not that ideal for the mechanics of the device itself. The pump ends up struggling to overcome the higher pressure—lowering the blood flow as a result. The slower the blood flows, the higher the risk of clot formation, so with elevated blood pressure, we are unnecessarily risking blood clots (definitely something we want to avoid at any cost). On the other hand, when the blood pressure is too low, the patient will experience dizziness and even fainting. As you see, we are in charge of artificially maintaining a very delicate balance.

During the first months of normal life outside of the hospital, our patients will report back to us for scheduled checkups. This allows us to monitor each individual case, adjusting and intervening wherever necessary. As you may imagine, doing so inside the hospital is much more convenient than helping our patients at home. When we are treating a patient in a BTD (bridge to decision) scenario, this period allows us to conduct further tests and diagnostics. The value of all these hospital visits cannot be understated, as the outcome will eventually decide the patient's potential viability for the heart transplant waiting list.

When the dust has settled, every question has been answered, every important detail has been cleared up (we now know if the patient is viable for a heart transplant or a long life with a steel heart), and we can safely start to decrease the number of scheduled hospital visits. In ideal situations, we will expect to see our patient every six to twelve months.

For the record, this is how we do things in our hospital (in Leuven, Belgium). Your country may have completely different requirements and schedules. Let's not forget that every patient and their medical history is quite different as well. Some will require a more frequent follow-up schedule; others will require less. We're all human, and it's all a matter of proper management of staff, patients, and schedules. We always try to optimize our procedures and protocols in order to allow a smooth and efficient system of follow-up for all our patients. The patient is our priority, and we will adjust ourselves to ensure every patient receives proper care and support.

Once you have been home for a few weeks with your heart pump, you will likely want to get out and live life! So a very important question comes to mind:

What activities are prohibited while living with an LVAD?

This is *the* question that most patients and family members usually ask us. Our patient wakes up with a shiny new piece of tech that is literally keeping them alive! It goes without saying that any patient is curious to know what they can and cannot do so as not to upset their new metallic best friend. Luckily, this list is quite short:

- No swimming
- No baths
- Never forget your blood-thinning medications
- No MRI machines

Swimming or being submerged in water wreaks havoc on the driveline's electrical connection. Aside from this, the skin around the driveline exit site can become soggy and swollen—giving bacteria a fighting chance to attach to the driveline and cause a nasty infection. So for the second time, please NO swimming and NO baths! How do we go about solving the problem of basic daily hygiene?

Luckily, there are special shower bags that allow patients to protect the driveline and control unit during showers. It keeps everything nice and dry, allowing you the pleasure of having a refreshing shower and a squeaky-clean body. Somewhere in the future, scientists and engineers will solve this problem. I'm very confident in this. For now, suffice it to say that a lack of bathing and swimming is definitely not a deal-breaker when doctors and technology have just given you a second chance to live fully.

Now let's dry off, blow dry our hair, and head over to the medicine cabinet. You already know the importance of blood thinning medication—we want to avoid the risks of blood clots at all costs. What about MRI? This important topic deserves a bit more explanation.

A magnetic resonance imaging scanner is a machine that uses extremely high magnetic fields to look inside a patient's body. If you're curious, a CT scan performs very similar functions using X-rays. Both methods have their pros and cons, and both are extremely useful in medicine. What makes the MRI so different?

You see, we're dealing with extremely strong magnetic fields. Sometimes ranging to 3 Tesla or even higher. To give you an idea of just how strong this is, consider that the earth's natural magnetic field is about 0.00005 Tesla. If you're curious about metal objects and the effect of MRI, turn to the internet! There are plenty of video's made by MRI technicians on this topic and posted online.

Before every MRI scan, a patient fills out an extensive questionnaire to determine if there are any metal parts present inside the body. Inside the MRI machine, you won't find any metal parts as well—any loose metallic object effectively becomes a live projectile that will be sucked into the machine at an incredibly high velocity and inevitably damage the patient who happens to be undergoing a scan at that critical moment.

As you remember from previous chapters, a heart pump is electro-magnetically driven, and the rotor levitates inside a magnetic field in order to make a frictionless and longer-lasting design. This tiny magnetic field of the LVAD is nothing compared to the gargantuan forces of the MRI machine. In other words, the MRI will stop the rotor of the heart pump as easily as an elephant would crush a fly.

Let's compare this MRI to a normal CT scan. This procedure can be done in as little as twenty seconds. An MRI is an entirely different beast. It's massive, slow, and takes a while to get up to speed. Meanwhile, the massive electromagnetic forces are constantly present while the machine is in operation. An MRI examination easily takes twenty minutes to be completed, and twenty minutes without an LVAD will kill you! So why bother to use a machine that needs so long to make images at all in medicine? Well, first of all, for certain pathologies, the image quality is superior. Second, magnetic waves are harmless to all humans, except LVAD patients, of course. The same is not true for X-rays. In high dosages, X-rays might cause mutations in your cells. So, there are strict rules on how much X-ray radiation a patient is allowed to absorb at any given time. Long story short, let's remember to avoid the MRI machine and focus on a healthy and productive lifestyle. Speaking of which . . .

Sports of any kind are incredibly healthy for anyone. What about heart-pump patients? We definitely advise doing sports, but with moderate levels of physical stress. For example, walking or riding a bicycle (electric or old-school) are absolutely wonderful activities for anyone living with a steel heart. We actively promote and encourage our patients to head out into the real world and pick up an active lifestyle.

When it comes to heavy physical efforts, this is where things are a bit more complicated. You see, regardless of all the technological improvements, the heart pump is programmed to work at a certain "fixed" amount of rotations per minute. In other words, the rotor of the pump is a bit "dumb". Every single minute a fixed amount of blood will flow from the left ventricle into the aorta. As you strain to push yourself to maximum effort, more and more blood will flow from the tiny veins of your muscles toward your heart—desperately gasping for fresh oxygen. The pump will have to deal with a greater demand for blood. Ideally, the heart pump would need to provide a higher flow, but as the RPM (rotations per minute) stays unchanged, very little additional flow is generated. Currently, there are no programmed algorithms inside the control unit that can increase the RPM in response to physical activity. So is any physical activity that is a tiny bit more demanding impossible?

No, as you push and strain yourself during heavy physical activities, your own heart will get stimulated to increase the blood flow in a completely natural way. Yes, even sick hearts that need an LVAD still have some potential to increase their output when the body demands it. So your heart pumps faster and stronger, increasing the blood flow in the systemic circulation. Great, now let's take advantage of the mighty power of the steel heart on top of that!

In the past, we tried to conduct experiments with increasing rates of blood flow inside an artificial heart pump, but unfortunately, the results were not at all promising. When we start increasing the amount of RMP inside our LVAD, this will have negative effects on our own natural heart. In essence the steel heart will start to deprive your own heart of enough blood to fully take advantage of the stronger and faster contractions. It's quite self-explanatory that this is a no-go for us. Hence the RMP of the heart pump remains fixed.

Some patients with incredibly poor heart function (bordering on zero) will somewhat benefit from a system with variable amounts of RPM. In studies, we found that they had a moderate increase in the total amount of blood that was pumped to the systemic circulation. Despite this, it was still in no way sufficient to facilitate any type of heavy physical effort.

As of today, this fixed amount of RMP (and blood flow) is working together with your natural heart function. It's a delicate biological and mechanical cooperation that allows the split of the blood flow across both hearts to work as one perfect system. Let's not screw it up, shall we?

What about contact sports then?

Unfortunately, this is not something we would recommend to any patient with a need for heavy doses of blood thinners. It is not recommended that patients with a heart pump play American football or get in the boxing ring. Don't worry, though, there's also good news: the most intimate contact sport is definitely allowed! This can sometimes be a challenge for men, due to obvious biological reasons—there needs to be ample blood flow to the penis. This requires a steady blood pressure, and this can sometimes be a bit of a deal breaker for some gentlemen. Luckily, there are medications that can help. Your doctor will have a much better idea of how to handle this delicate situation. So don't be afraid to ask them; you won't be the first to pop the question.

Note that intimacy does become a bit of a different game with an LVAD. The pump is always connected to the controller and batteries or the charging cable. Some patients have reported that the charging cable of the control unit gets in the way, but very soon patients learned to navigate this obstacle in the best way possible. If you want proof of this, consider that some young men (with an artificial heart pump) have already become proud fathers! This fact alone wipes the floor of the taboo that sex with a heart pump is impossible. When it comes to women, the situation is unfortunately different. Although intimate life is not an issue, a pregnancy during LVAD is contraindicated due to the high risks to both the mother and the fetus. You might think, "Accidents happen all the time." Indeed they do, and in literature there are definitely a few reports of successful pregnancies during LVAD support. But let me be very clear, I definitely advise you not to get pregnant while living with an LVAD.

What about driving? This is also not a problem. After each heart surgery in Belgium, you're not legally allowed to drive until you have been given a green light by your doctor. This will usually happen somewhere between four to six weeks after your operation. At that point you can request a medical certificate that allows you to put the pedal to the metal. The same rules apply to patients who have just been out-fitted with their brand-new heart pump. Most of our patients today happily drive around without a care in the world. And some of them even conveniently use their 12V power output to top off their batteries. Yes, this is also possible!

However, some potential complications to the health of a patient with a steel heart can result in a temporary ban from public roads. This might include a stroke or seizures that occurred, for example. In some cases, you will even be asked to take some additional medical tests before you can receive a new driver's license and be welcome on the road again.

When it comes to traveling, this is also not a problem for our patients. But remember, it's definitely a good idea to go to places that have access to electrical power. You need an access point to charge your batteries, so please don't go out into the Brazilian jungle looking for new, undiscovered species of spiders just yet! Most of our patients are quite successful at traveling. One or two weeks away to a foreign country with family and friends is definitely possible. Before you start packing your suitcases, let's take some time to consider Doug Casey's "6 P's"—proper planning prevents piss-poor performance!

First, you'll need to have a chat with the VAD coordinator. Aside from providing you with helpful advice, they will also instruct you on some very often overlooked matters as you're planning to travel abroad. For example, we will always provide you with contact information of the nearest hospital where "steel heart" specialists can be found. Remember, regardless of your travel destination, it's always important to remember that not every hospital is qualified to receive and treat patients with an LVAD. Now, as we have these matters sorted, let's move on to traveling itself.

You will need certain certificates that you'll show to the security staff in the airports, as well as to the staff of the airline of your choice. As you may already imagine, all that metal inside the heart pump and control unit will trigger the metal detectors at the airport. The medical certificates will make your security check a breeze. Next on the list are your batteries. Always take a spare and always think about an access point for charging them. Now that you have these matters sorted, I wish you a bon voyage!

As we head into the next chapter, it's worth noting that if you are one of the lucky patients who made it onto the list of heart transplants, sadly your world exploration will have to wait. You see, as soon as a viable donor heart is available, it's a race against the clock to get you into the operating theater as soon as humanly possible. It's quite self-explanatory that we can't do this while you're rubbing coconut oil onto your stomach under the tropical sun in Hawaii. For the sake of your life, you will have to stay at home for now!

CHAPTER 7

DANGERS OF LIVING WITH A HEART PUMP

"Hearts will never be practical until they can be made unbreakable."
—*The Wizard of Oz*

THIS QUOTE IS QUITE RELEVANT TO OUR LONG-TERM heart pumps. Every machine, no matter how well it's made, can eventually break down. Many companies today practice the well-known principles of *planned obsolescence*. We are "stimulated" to go out and buy shiny new stuff every few years to keep the economy going. I'm delighted to say that these nefarious practices don't apply to our heart pumps. On the contrary, we aim to design and build these amazing devices to be as long-lasting as physically possible! How long exactly? Try ten, fifteen years (sometimes even longer) of carefree life. Imagine an engine working nonstop for more than ten years. This is a truly amazing result that medical science has achieved in just a few decades.

Before you rejoice at the prospect of your second life, let's take a moment to cover all the potential risks that patients with a steel heart may run into at some point in life. Most of these risks are not associated with the function of the heart pump itself. These are rather side effects of life with a heart pump. We'll focus on these side effects first before covering potential issues with the pump unit itself.

BLEEDING ISSUES

Every heart surgery has a risk of potential bleeding issues. We are operating on major blood vessels and the ventricles—the risk is quite real. As we wrap up every surgical procedure, we meticulously check for the absence of bleeding. After we make sure that everything is okay, we will leave a few tiny tubes inside the patient's chest. These tubes will allow any blood left after the surgery to exit the patient's body. If for some reason we encounter heavy bleeding, we will immediately conduct a reintervention to rectify this situation.

Fast-forward a few days. Now the danger of post-operative internal bleeding has subsided. However, as you remember, the patient now requires special blood thinners to accommodate the new heart pump. Without these medications, the feared blood clots might rear their ugly heads inside the LVAD! This presents us with another challenge—the risk of internal bleeding in other areas. You might not know this, but the heart pump lowers some clotting factor in the blood. It's called the *von Willebrand factor*—a large protein that's always present in our blood. This protein is responsible for producing blood clots in areas where our blood vessels are damaged—essentially ensuring that any type of bleeding stops as soon as possible. This protein needs a certain length to function properly, but it can also not be too long, or it would cause clot formation in healthy blood vessels. Complex right? But our body has a solution.

Let's dive deep into our cardiovascular system to see what happens. As we travel across our bloodstream, we can observe a peculiar phenomenon; inside our blood vessels where the blood is flowing at a steady pace, this von Willebrand protein gets stretched out if it becomes too long and eventually gets cut into smaller pieces by another protein (called ADAMTS-13). Compare it with putting a string of rope in a river. If there is no flow of water, the rope will just sink to the bottom and be a ball of rope. The faster the river flows, the more the rope will get stretched. The rope is the von Willebrand factor, and ADAMTS-13 is cutting the rope as it gets stretched. In our blood vessels, the flow rate is quite constant, and thousands and thousands of years of evolution have balanced the production and cutting of von Willebrand factor in our blood vessels to perfection.

When we are dealing with the fast rotor of the steel heart, things look quite different. As you remember, the rotor is spinning at a whopping speed of up to twenty thousand rotations per minute in some pumps! As the blood flow is sped up by the rotor, the von Willebrand proteins get stretched out more. The rope is not in a nice quiet river anymore, but in a raging white-water creek in the Alaskan mountains! These von Willebrand proteins cannot handle the harsh reality of this very rapid blood flow, and they are cut into smaller pieces than usual (because they are stretched to the limit). These smaller pieces are no longer able to stop a bleeding event. Aside from the blood-thinning medication that the patient already takes, this natural mechanical mutation of the von Willebrand proteins can increase the risks of internal bleeding.

So patients with an LVAD have a higher risk of bleeding events. Which types of bleeding do we see most often, you wonder? Well, we see it inside the nose, stomach, and gastrointestinal system, or even inside the brain. An innocent nosebleed is definitely not a deal-breaker. The others are, of course, much more serious! These bleeding events can become life-threatening if not addressed properly. After all, the last thing we want to see is a patient with permanent brain damage due to a bleeding in the brain. Unfortunately, strokes are a real threat to LVAD patients, and it is one of the issues we need to keep working on. A stroke can be lethal or have major consequences for the quality of life of our patients.

RISKS OF THROMBOSES

Now you know about the risks of having blood that is too thin, let's look at the other side of the equation. What happens when the blood becomes too thick? Again, we enter the risk territory. This is why it's always a good practice to maintain the delicate balance of the coagulation state as we go through life with a heart pump. Just like the plate of porridge inside the home of the three bears, our blood can't be too thin or too thick. It has to be just right!

As you now know, when the blood is not anticoagulated enough (when it becomes too thick), the risk of blood clots forming inside the heart pump is never too far away! These clots love to form in places where our blood is flowing at a much slower rate. Let's dive into our heart pump and try to find these danger zones. As you know, the heart pump rotor is always spinning at a constant rate. The blood will organize itself inside the pump body to flow in the most efficient way possible.

Let's compare this blood flow to a river. In the middle of our river, the water will always run faster than at the shoreline. Remember those physics classes from high school? Yes, now you need them! For the sake of this simple example, let's imagine that our river will have a constant steady supply of water to all the zones. The result is very simple; both the fast zone (in the middle of the river) and the slow zone (at the shoreline) will be dealing with a constant stream of water at any given time. So, the flow is highly organized and stays that way, fast in the middle area, slow at the shore. Simple, right?

The same tends to happen inside the heart pump body. When the flow is constant, there are areas where the blood is flowing nice and quickly and then there are areas where the blood likes to slow down and linger for a while. These slow areas have the highest risk of developing a clot! Now, it's quite self-explanatory that we cannot just clean these areas at will, as the heart pump lives happily inside our patient's chest. Luckily, the engineers have found a brilliant solution.

The control unit of the heart pump is programmed to perform a wash-out cycle. Every two seconds the rotor of the heart pump will slow down and speed back up again. This mechanical trick ensures that the constant flow of blood is interrupted. No more steady pattern of quick and slow moving blood. This sudden change in RPMs results in a turbulent flow, washing out all the slow, lingering blood inside the heart pump. As a result, the risk of blood clotting inside the pump is drastically reduced.

It's interesting to mention that the wash-out motion of the rotor also creates a measurable difference in blood pressure—an artificial pulse. The absolute value of this pressure difference is minor, and the patient won't even notice it. Common blood pressure equipment is also not sensitive enough for this task. We have to rely on intra-arterial blood pressure monitors to "sense" this pulse. These machines are quite rare beasts. They live only in the intensive care units of the hospital.

Let's take a moment to analyze a worst-case scenario—a pump thrombosis. This happens when blood clots suddenly appear inside the heart pump. There are a few important signs that a patient must know about. Someday, this information may save your life! Often, the first sign of a pump thrombosis is an unmistakable red discoloration of the urine. Whenever a patient sees this phenomenon, it's time to visit the hospital as soon as humanly possible. Why exactly?

You see, hemolysis (the destruction of red blood cells) related to a pump thrombosis can permanently damage the patient's kidneys. As if this wasn't enough, if for any reason whatsoever a blood clot sitting inside the pump suddenly dislodges and starts traveling throughout the bloodstream, it *will* inflict damage to the patient's organs, with the possibility of creating a major stroke if it reaches the brain. As a cherry on top, further blood clotting can interfere with the rotor of the LVAD itself—to the point of a complete failure.

So what can we do if a cloth starts to develop inside the pump? Every patient is unique, and every situation is different. As a first line of defense, we could try to clear up blood clots using special medication that breaks down clots. If this step is futile, we will need to replace the heart pump entirely. It's quite self-explanatory that this is indeed a quite serious operation. Again, let's remember to maintain the delicate balance between thick and thin blood—it has to be just right!

RISK OF SUCTION

As we covered all the control unit's alarms, the *suction alarm* is quite important—to the point of covering it in a bit more detail here. As you remember, sometimes the pump's inflow cannula can come a bit too close to the walls of the left ventricle. The strong suction force will grab the side of the ventricle, and blood flow will temporarily be halted. As a result of this unnatural disturbance, the controller will immediately decrease the rotor's speed and allow the inflow cannula to naturally detach itself from the inside wall of the left ventricle.

This happens more commonly than you may think. Sometimes we see patients with multiple suction alarms firing off every single day. Naturally, this is not a fun experience for the patient! Not by a long shot. You see, as the pump grabs the inner wall of the left ventricle, it can cause a so-called *ventricular arrhythmia*. In other words, this event will disrupt your natural heart rhythm. As if this wasn't enough, the lack of blood flow through our LVAD (as it grabs the inner wall of the left ventricle instead of pumping blood) will cause discomfort to our patient.

Any suction alarm we encounter presents a new mystery. In every case we will do our very best to find the cause of this issue and solve it once and for all. In most cases a suction alarm will be the result of a too-high dose of diuretic medication. Diuretics decrease the amount of water in your blood. This can lead to a lower filling state of the cardiovascular system and thus the left ventricle. The smaller the ventricle, the higher the chance that the cannula will grab the ventricular wall. When we reduce this diuretic medication dose to more normal levels, the issue will be solved, and the patient can be on their way back home.

Since every patient is unique, sometimes we have cases of suction alarms that are the result of an irregular heart rhythm. As we are dealing with an aberrant heart rhythm, the right ventricle tends to contract in a less efficient way than normal. The result of this is less blood flow to the lungs and eventually less blood arriving in the left atrium and ventricle. But our heart pump has a fixed speed, right? So as the right ventricle struggles with the supply of blood to the left side, the heart pump pumps out more blood than arrives, in the end draining the left ventricle empty and creating suction.

But wait, was a suction event in itself not a cause of aberrant heart rhythm? Yes, you have it damn right. It goes without saying that this event mobilizes a small army of doctors as we go about conducting a proper investigation and determining the cause and effect of this matter. Every patient is unique and requires our full attention.

RISK OF INFECTIONS

As you already know, an intact skin barrier is the best protection against infections. As the driveline exits the patient's abdomen, the integrity of the skin is compromised and the driveline itself becomes a risk zone for infections. This is why we spend so much attention on educating our patients about proper disinfection and care of this highly important lifeline to your LVAD. No matter how well you may follow the procedures, this driveline is still one of the biggest risks for developing infections. It's quite self-explanatory that the longer a patient is living with a heart pump, the higher this risk becomes.

If an infection does occur, we sometimes can see it crawling alongside the length of the cable, digging deeper and deeper into the patient's body. As this occurs, we will need to enlist the help of antibiotics. They can slow down this process (and sometimes stop it in its tracks). However, they won't be able to heal this infection entirely. Why exactly? Bacteria are tenacious little critters! They love to nestle on the surface of the driveline and form a kind of *biofilm* (a type of artificially constructed protective environment that helps them survive and thrive). If we are dealing with a serious infection, our treatment will, in part, depend on the scenario of implantation of the LVAD. Remember, every scenario is different. Hence, every single patient will require a fully bespoke treatment strategy. Let's look at a few examples.

When our heavily infected patient happens to be in a BTT scenario (bridge to transplant), we will consider an urgent heart transplantation.

During DT (destination therapy), we will consider a surgical cleaning of the cable. As an added precaution, we can even change the trajectory of the driveline inside the patient's abdomen. During this procedure, we will sometimes opt to move the driveline inside the abdomen and wrap the fatty tissue (the omentum) that sits there around the cable. This is quite a common practice in medicine in general when we're dealing with notoriously tenacious infections.

You may not know this, but the omentum (fatty tissue of the abdomen) is an ideal substance for solving the problem of infections. It contains a plethora of tiny blood vessels. Thanks to these blood vessels, fighting infection becomes a lot easier. Our blood is home to white blood cells that love nothing more than hunting down and gobbling up all the foreign invaders, such as our tenacious bacteria. Great news for the patient! Horrible news for the tiny critters.

If the infection is so severe and widespread that even our body can't handle it properly, we can always remove and replace the infected driveline and LVAD in their entirety. Yes, sadly, sometimes the infection can reach the LVAD itself. During DT (destination therapy), it's important to eliminate all the bacteria and their protective biofilms. This is why we will sometimes choose such a heavy intervention. Besides, sometimes our patients still have an old version of a heart pump. In this case they will definitely benefit from a much-needed upgrade.

Let's keep in mind that we are talking about a very serious and heavy surgery. It's important that our patient is strong and healthy to handle (and recover from) this long and difficult procedure.

Nowadays, the majority of admissions to the hospital for LVAD patients are due to infections. Remember, if you're reading these words and there's a heart pump buzzing inside your chest right now, keep your driveline squeaky clean at all times! You have been warned!

Another type of infection we have to be very careful about is *endocarditis*. Again, let's explain the term before we dig deeper. The endocardium is the inner layer of your heart, and the suffix *-itis* means infection. So the two terms combined indicate an infection of the inner layer of your heart. Most commonly the valves of your heart will be infected by bacteria when you have endocarditis. As with myocarditis, it can happen to any one of us. Yet artificial heart valves or any foreign material living in your heart has a greater risk of becoming infected. Indeed, the bacteria that love to colonize your driveline also love these islands of foreign material inside your heart. How do the little creeps get there, you wonder? Not through the driveline, but through our bloodstream.

You see, bacteria love blood, rich in oxygen and nutrition, so whenever they see an entrance, they will try to dive in. Luckily our blood is well guarded by the white blood cells, killing them rapidly. But when they manage to reach one of these islands of foreign material, they might settle in their biofilm, making it impossible for your body to fight them off. Oftentimes, endocarditis can only be solved by surgery, in which we have to remove all the infected tissue. These operations are heavy and high-risk, so let's try to avoid that, shall we? Whenever we give an opportunity to bacteria to dive deep into your bloodstream, we will boost your body's defenses by giving antibiotics. Wait, why would we ever give bacteria an opportunity to dive into your body? Well, a colonoscopy, dental care, and any surgical procedure bring breaches to your body's outer defense layer against bacteria. So, whenever you have to undergo such a procedure, be sure to take some antibiotics beforehand. How long and which ones? Your doctor will tell you but be damn sure to take them!

RISK OF RIGHT VENTRICLE FAILURE

We already know that the steel heart supports the left ventricle. As the LVAD is continuously working, we observed a peculiar side effect; the resistance of the blood flow inside our lungs becomes significantly lower! You already know what happens to the right ventricle in this situation—thanks to the lack of blood flow resistance, the right ventricle will have a much easier time pumping blood across our pulmonary circulation. Most patients are quite happy with this arrangement, especially patients who suffer from myocardial infarction. As you may remember, the left ventricle is the beefed-up muscular part of your heart. The right ventricle is the skinny dude riding along on the hard work of the left ventricle. Obviously, the left ventricle needs more blood supply, and in a myocardial infarction, it often is harder hit than the right ventricle. This simply means that as the LVAD is assisting the left ventricle, the fruits of this mechanical labor also spill over to a better (and easier) function of the right ventricle. We are indeed happy with this arrangement!

This situation changes drastically from the moment we are dealing with a non-ischemic cause of heart failure—in this case, both ventricles will have life-threatening, severely reduced function. Now the pump assisting the left side is also helping the right ventricle by lowering the resistance over the lung vessels. Victory, you might think! Not always. As the left side is pumping more blood through the systemic circulation, more blood is coming to the right ventricle. So the gains of lower resistance are sometimes erased by having to pump more blood to the lungs. Sometimes we will even see the right ventricle struggling more and more as time progresses. In essence, right ventricle failure is clearly visible on the horizon! During DT (destination therapy), this is unfortunately the worst-case scenario. In the majority of cases, the patient will arrive at the hospital experiencing similar symptoms that plagued them before the LVAD implantation. You could opt for an additional heart pump for the right ventricle, but this is done only in very rare cases. Another option would be to replace the heart completely with a totally artificial heart. In some countries these amazing machines are used, but in Belgium we don't have them available. This is why we go out of our way to perform thorough patient screening before considering a heart pump implantation procedure. Heart failure is already a quite severe disease. Heart failure with a steel heart is definitely even worse.

RISK OF PUMP FAILURE

Before we proceed any further, let's clarify one important detail. When we're talking about "pump failure," we literally mean the primary failure of the heart pump itself. We are not talking about potential complications that may surface as a result of a blood clot inside the pump body. As you already know by now, when a large blood clot forms inside the pump body, the rotor will jam, and the heart pump will stop working. Naturally, this doesn't mean that the heart pump itself was faulty or broken in any way. The pump worked flawlessly, and the cause of the malfunction was a blood clot. Let's remember to monitor the blood and keep an eye on the correct medication at the correct time.

The reason why the above-mentioned paragraph may sound a bit harsh, is because this is something we struggle with explaining to many of our patients. Very often during a complication (the risks of complications are *always* present during any surgical procedure), patients tend to search for something to blame. Coincidently, the LVAD itself is a prime candidate for venting any anger, resentment, and suspicion.

The same goes for infections of the driveline. The infection is a complication that can occur in any patient with any type of cable. So, it is not because the driveline is broken or has a manufacturing fault that the infection occurs. It's not a defect of the driveline that causes the driveline to infect. It is the breached skin barrier that is to blame.

In some cases, though, the heart pump can fail. In the next part, we will mention failures that occurred. Don't panic if you read this. Many of the issues have been resolved. As we covered the history of the steel hearts, you already know that the current designs are much safer and more reliable than the units we used just twenty years ago. We are insanely lucky that the technology keeps evolving and the insatiable hunger of engineers and designers is never satisfied with the current reality. Even with these current pump designs, there are always risks of mechanical failure. In the end, an LVAD is a device, and no device is 100 percent failure-free. In recent literature there are some surveys looking at the rates of technical issues of the LVAD and its so-called peripherals (the controller, the batteries, the driveline). They found that issues with these devices are not so uncommon, but many of these are related to the peripherals that you can easily replace (a battery or a controller). Most of these issues are also not endangering the patient. But some issues with the device and its peripherals are more serious and deserve some attention. We will address them now.

In 2022, a certain type of pump was taken off the market due to risks of malfunction—in some cases the pump could come to a complete standstill without restart. We have seen some batches of these pumps reach a 30 percent risk of a complete standstill. As a precaution, the manufacturer recommended preventively replacing these units.

A problem that might arise is the so-called ESD (*electrostatic discharge*) event. Indeed, the electric shock you sometimes get from touching an object that has static electricity could interfere with your LVAD, even leading to a full stop. When this was first noted, our patients were taught precautionary measures to avoid electrostatic discharges.

Other problems also arise from the motion of your inner parts. As you go about your day, your lungs inflate and deflate, your diaphragm moves up and down, and your abdominal muscles contract as you walk. Also your biological heart will conduct its normal function of contraction and relaxation. So much motion! This motion translates to the LVAD. Over time, these repeated movements can start to cause wear and tear of the LVAD. One issue was with the outflow graft. The graft connecting the pump part of the LVAD to the aorta could start to twist. That twist obstructed the outflow graft. An unexpected issue for the manufacturer! The quick fix was a special clip to prevent twisting of the graft, and newer models had a different connection of the graft to the pump to eliminate the problem permanently.

The driveline is the second victim of this continuous motion inside your body. You can imagine what these mechanical forces do to a driveline over the long term. You may already guess that after a few years, the driveline can start showing signs of normal wear and tear, and it's only natural that we will start seeing potential defects. In older designs a crack in a special protecting sheet could create a power loss to the LVAD when connected to a grounded power source. This was called the *short-to-shield phenomenon*. Again, a quick fix in those cases was to use an ungrounded power source, and in newer designs of LVADs, this phenomenon is resolved entirely. Inside the driveline, there are three electrical wires going to the LVAD. Each one has a backup wire, so in total six wires are inside the driveline. When two wires break and make contact, they can also create a shortcut. This is called the *wire-to-wire phenomenon*. Again, engineers will try everything they can to fix this as it occurs, but sometimes the defect is beyond their reach.

Although materials improve and become more resilient, physical wear and tear still applies to even the newest designs, and they are still not indestructible marvels of technology. At some point, electrical wiring inside the driveline can break down, even in today's designs of LVADs.

We may naturally ask ourselves, "Why not simply replace the driveline?" This is easier said than done. You see, the pump and cable are actually one, inseparable unit. Replacing the driveline means replacing the pump as well, and that is a heavy surgical procedure! In the past, engineers tried to create a separate connection where the driveline simply plugs into the LVAD, but we quickly discovered that this opens a whole new can of worms. This design needlessly subjects our patient to an even higher risk than the driveline issues. The connection between the driveline and the pump became a liability with a higher probability of failure than the cable failing due to continuous motion. As you may imagine, we quickly abandoned this idea.

When a patient is waiting for a heart transplant, it's safe to say that they will almost never run into issues with their heart pump due to wear and tear. Most of these patients will happily receive a heart transplant within two to three years at most (although a few years seem like an eternity when you're on the waiting list for a donor heart). During this time, their steel heart will usually work flawlessly. The chance that you will see a UFO in the night sky is higher than a heart pump suddenly stopping or breaking down. Yes, this is how confident we are about the quality of modern LVADs.

What about our patients in the DT (destination therapy) scenario? These are the people who are living with a steel heart until the day they step through the tunnel of eternal light. Will their LVAD be equally reliable and long-lasting? Short answer—yes.

You see, most patients in the DT scenario will not live long enough to experience mechanical pump failure. It may be harsh to read, but for most patients, it is a true statement. Let's remember that patients in the DT scenario are not candidates for a heart transplant, and this is usually due to other health issues or older age. We are all susceptible to the ravages of time, and over time, even the healthiest body will simply start to deteriorate. This is perfectly normal.

Using a heart pump, we aim to improve the patient's quality of life and prolong a satisfying life for as long as humanly possible. Sadly, this period cannot currently be measured in decades but only years. Currently around 60 percent of DT patients cross the five-year threshold with the help of their heart pump. Common mechanical pump failures usually occur only after many more years of flawless operation.

As we are constantly honing our skills, improving our methods, and working with much better technology, we expect to see many more DT patients cross the five-year barrier. So at some point in the future device failure in DT setting might become a prominent problem. Needless to say that technology and medicine will also progress. I'm confident we will have solutions when that time comes.

So what exactly happens when a steel heart fails? Contrary to popular belief, when a heart pump experiences an electrical failure, it doesn't always translate into an immediate death sentence for our patient! Usually the sequence of events starts with quite loud and noticeable alarm tones—the control unit will detect an electrical problem and without any hesitation notify the patient. Sometimes we can even use a few nifty tricks to prevent a heart pump from stalling completely. This can be achieved with the help of a special type of controller.

When the electrical pump failure occurs in the body of a young and fit patient, it's quite self-explanatory that we will do our very best to replace the entire unit (pump and driveline). An alternative strategy could be to go for an urgent transplantation. Currently, more and more steel heart patients find themselves in the category of DT. But not every DT patient is still young and fit. So, we do our very best to discuss all the risks and instruct the patients on the potential courses of action during a pump failure event. After all, when you're on your way to the emergency room, it helps to be well-informed and know what to expect next. Some patients are happy with the additional quality time they had with the LVAD and don't want any more invasive procedures. Remember Geraldine, the granny? She is one of them. Let's see how her story ended.

When Geraldine went home with her brand-new LVAD, she was living with her husband at home. The first three years passed by without any problem. Her LVAD worked flawlessly, and she enjoyed every day with her husband, children, and grandchildren around her. But then the trouble started. Her husband suddenly died, and Geraldine herself was diagnosed with leukemia a few months later. Determined to see her grandchildren grow up, she went for full-on chemotherapy, with success! A year later she had tackled this disease, managing the household on her own.

But now, in her eighties, age is starting to catch up with her, and at the age of eighty-two she has to accept the fact that living alone in the big house is no longer an option. She moves to an elderly care home where she is the talk of the month when she arrives. The first ever resident with an LVAD! The staff was a bit apprehensive to have her under their care, but Geraldine hadn't lost her charm and sense of humor. Very soon she was embraced as a normal resident in her new home. Geraldine is smart enough to know that this would, in fact, be her last home, her final chapter in life. A few years later, the pump controller started to give strange alarms.

Engineers of the LVAD manufacturer tried every trick they had up their sleeve, but unfortunately, it didn't work. From time to time her pump would stop all of a sudden and restart after a while. In the readouts from the pump data, we learned that it might be seconds to a minute before the pump restarted. Geraldine's own heart condition was reassessed. You remember the bridge to recovery (BTR) scenario? Well, imagine that Geraldine's heart recovered from her myocardial infarction. Then we could maybe decommission the LVAD and let her enjoy the rest of her life without this faulty pump.

But wait, you said she didn't want any more surgical procedures? And if you take all the risks to explant the LVAD, why not replace it while you are there? Well, if we would decommission her LVAD we wouldn't bring her to the OR and open her chest again. No, we would simply put a stent in the outflow graft between the LVAD and the aorta to occlude this graft. This can be done under local anesthesia with only a little cut in the groin. We would navigate the stent through the arterial vascular system (just like we do with a catheter-mounted pump) and position it in the outflow graft. Then we would stop the LVAD, cut the driveline some ten centimeters (about four inches) before the driveline exit site, and bury it deep under the skin to prevent future infections.

The LVAD would still be in her body but not work any longer. So why not just stop the LVAD and cut the cable? If we did that, the outflow graft would still be open, allowing blood to flow back from the aorta into the ventricle. Normally this doesn't happen because the LVAD generates pressure in the graft, directing the blood *to* the aorta, *away* from the left ventricle. If the LVAD is stopped, blood will flow *away* from the aorta *to* the left ventricle. Even a perfectly healthy ventricle can't handle this, and you wouldn't last a day. So if the LVAD is stopped, the outflow graft has to be occluded.

Unfortunately for Geraldine, her heart function hasn't recovered anywhere near a level we could consider this option. Her pump stops become more frequent, and the idea that her life is now in the hands of a faulty device is troubling her mind. Also, the nursing staff in the care home is worried. What can they do if her LVAD stops for minutes and doesn't restart? For the VAD coordinator, to whom Geraldine has become a third grandmother, it is clear that we have to bring her to the hospital. Geraldine feels safer in the hospital, the staff in the nursing home can take a breather, and we have ample time to discuss the situation with her.

After careful consideration, Geraldine is admitted to the hospital, feeling relieved that her problem is being taken seriously. On the other side, she's feeling anxious, knowing that all the options are quickly running out. The time to worry was cut short when the next morning she passed away in her bed. During her sleep, the LVAD stopped and sadly didn't restart anymore. For ten long years Geraldine's steel heart kept her alive and smiling. Sadly, everyone's story will eventually come to an end, and at some time we will all have to step through the tunnel of light.

Before you start to worry about the longevity of Geraldine's LVAD, it's important to make two quick remarks. One, the device she received is now no longer used. It was a second-generation unit that is no longer being implanted today. Chances are high that you already have the third-generation device that will work even longer. Two, we have seen many patients living much longer with flawlessly working second-generation devices. As you may already expect, ten years is definitely *not* the maximum lifespan of these devices.

RISK OF AORTIC VALVE INSUFFICIENCY

An LVAD sucks blood from the left ventricle and sends it straight to the aorta. The outflow graft connects to the aorta, usually 5 to 7 cm above the aortic valve. This creates a peculiar situation where the blood pressure is pushing on the aortic valve from the completely opposite side. As this continues for years on end, all that extra pressure can cause the aortic valve to leak. That is why we replace or repair the valve during the implantation of an LVAD if we know aortic insufficiency is present. We have covered this in detail in the surgical procedure.

Now let's imagine this scenario. Our patient has a steel heart, and after a few years we start to notice valve leakage. Luckily, in most cases these leaks are rather limited in their severity, to the point of causing no observable health issues or even minor discomfort. Of course, there are some cases where this is different. This means we will need to evaluate the overall health condition of our patient. How fit and healthy are they? What's their general life expectancy? After answering more of these serious questions, we will determine the correct course of action and roll up our sleeves to help our patient further.

As you remember, for the sake of our patient's health, it's vital to use the least-invasive surgical methods at our disposal. For example, we can install a new valve using the femoral arteries (in the groin area). If you're curious, this is called the TAVI or TAVR procedure. First, we will fold the biological valve and use catheters to transport this folded valve through the femoral arteries directly to the aortic valve. Once there, we unfold this biological valve and push the old one to the side. Now our patient has a brand-new, shiny, and perfectly functioning aortic valve.

As you can imagine, this is but a short explanation of a quite complex procedure. The reality is not that simple. The TAVI valves are designed to replace calcified valves, so in essence valves with poor opening function. They are not designed to replace leaking valves. In fact, the calcification of the old valve is actually a quite useful surface where the new valve can gain better support. As if this isn't complicated enough, the new valve is guided by special metal wires that enter the left ventricle itself (where our LVAD is busy sucking up all the blood and pumping it straight to the aorta). We have to be extremely careful not to damage the inflow cannula or the rotor of our pump. It's no wonder that this delicate procedure is often reserved for patients who are deemed too weak to go to conventional surgery.

When our patient can physically handle a heart surgery, we can sometimes combine two procedures into one. We will replace the biological artificial valve together with the steel heart itself. Why? As the years go by, valve leakage can cause great discomfort to our patient. Coincidentally, if we notice issues with the LVAD (or when a new and safer design of a heart pump becomes available), we can kill two birds with one stone and solve both issues with just one surgical procedure. Remember, any heart surgery carries a certain degree of risk. This means we will always approach every unique case from all possible sides and choose the best, safest, and least invasive method possible.

CHAPTER 8

A LOOK AT OUR LVAD PROGRAM

BY NOW WE HAVE COVERED SO MUCH IMPORTANT MATE-rial! You are quite well informed about all the intricacies of our heart, as well as all the advancements in the field of LVADs. If by now your new knowledge can't impress your in-laws during Christmas dinner, I would consider this book a failure. All humor aside, it's important to always keep in mind that behind every medical story, there are real patients—real people living with their steel hearts—and each person has their personal story and quite unforgettable experiences.

This chapter looks beyond the medicine. As you might imagine, dealing with such a special care requires more than just well considered medical protocols and procedures. It requires a strategy combining all aspects of care. Not only is this incredibly interesting, but it also gives us an insider's look that simply cannot be found anywhere else. Needless to say that the VAD coordinator plays an essential role here. And how did they manage to improve our care over the years? By listening to the patients. People who are alive thanks to the help of an LVAD are quite rare, so it's incredibly interesting (and therapeutic) to listen to their side of the story.

Most of our patients (and their families) don't know any people who walk through life with their steel heart assisting them every second of every day. New patients feel quite alone and misunderstood. Yes, there is, of course, a small army of professional doctors, nurses, and VAD coordinators to help patients find their groove, but sadly, the real world exists outside the hospital walls. For us, it's quite important to help our patients every step of the way—in this case also psychologically.

We have taken the time to set up communities where patients can reach out to each other. Aside from these groups, we also maintain quite an active social media presence. It goes without saying that not everything you hear online should be taken at face value. Still, social media is a great tool to connect patients and let them bloom and settle back into a happy and fulfilling life. Besides, we are social creatures—we like to be understood, and we like to reach out to people who share our similarities. The same goes for our patients. We work hard to ensure every patient can keep in touch with us and with other patients as well.

Every year we host a dinner party for our patients and their partners. One of our LVAD patients happens to be a restaurant owner. We owe him a great degree of gratitude and generously took him up on his offer to hold a few of our annual meetings in his restaurant.

Such an event is always a warm and pleasant experience for every attendee. It's an informal and casual way to allow patients, doctors, and VAD coordinators to converse and mingle outside the confines of the hospital walls. You really notice how everyone enjoys this evening, being in the companionship of people who had to tackle the same obstacles in life. Also, the partners who come along to this dinner cannot be ignored. Their lives change drastically as well, as they have to adjust their lifestyle when their partner becomes equipped with a steel heart.

Some of our patients even receive special training to become formal *experts by experience*. This idea was developed in our hospital in the dialysis department. But the concept goes wider than only our hospital. So who are these experts by experience? Usually these are people with a (chronic) illness that changed the very nature of their daily life. They are the best point of reference for our new patients who have just been stuck with similar life-altering diagnoses.

So, in 2022 we started the expert by experience selection program in our hospital with the help of the charity that supports this program. After information rounds, interviews, and several meetings, we selected six patients and one of the patient's partners to become these so-called experts by experience. In this group we found people who were still living with a steel heart and people who already underwent heart transplants. Now all of them give proper guidance to our new patients, informing, supporting, and boosting their morale. All of them (including the partner of one of the patients) were thoroughly educated and coached by our team.

The expert by experience education is quite unique. It teaches the important aspects of medical secrecy, as well as certain professional listening and communication techniques. Although a treasure chest of knowledge themselves, these people are always welcome to speak with our specialists as well. Let's not forget that meeting new LVAD patients can be quite emotional events for the experts themselves. After every meeting they have with a new patient, we will also have a quick debrief with the expert to check how things went. In our practice, we have to be as thorough as possible.

When a new patient is implanted with a new heart pump, their VAD coordinator will advise them to speak with someone in a similar situation—an expert by experience. Naturally, we will do our best to find the best person that fits the social and medical needs of our patient. Ideally a potential DT (destination therapy) patient can speak to one of the experts beforehand. In doing so, the DT patient can take the information from the expert into his or her decision process regarding the LVAD implantation.

As of today, this system of peer support is working very well, and we cannot be more grateful to our experts because of it.

During the course of this book we have met a few patients already. Now would be a good moment to check in on them again.

The very first patient that we met was Michael. He was struck by a massive myocardial infarction on the golf course and first received an ECMO as a short-term pump. A week later this was followed by an

LVAD implantation. Michael has a quite favorable recollection of his LVAD period. He was able to adapt swiftly to the new reality of living with an LVAD. He sometimes referred to it with the quote: "Me and my LVAD." He appreciated the LVAD as a kind of buddy, a friend always on his side supporting him (in a hemodynamic way, at least). Nevertheless, he was quite happy when the long-awaited heart transplant arrived. Now he is enjoying his life intensely, fully appreciating that he really was given a second chance at life!

Not everyone makes such a swift adaptation to life with an LVAD. I still remember a man in his late fifties who received an LVAD. Despite an uneventful recovery after surgery and nothing but good test results upon every check-up, he wasn't happy with his LVAD. After the implantation he couldn't sleep anymore, he claimed.

But, Steven, you are a cardiac surgeon, why do you bother about his sleep? Well, LVADs are still such a new technology that we keep a close eye on all complaints of our patients. On one hand, we don't want to miss out on complications that we didn't know about, and on the other hand we want to guide the referral process to other specialists. You see, the last thing we want is an unaware doctor ordering an MRI for an LVAD patient, not knowing he *will* kill the patient inside the MRI machine. Nor do we want a surgeon stopping all anticoagulants for seven days (just to be sure the effect has worn off) for back surgery and along the way completely clot the LVAD. By doing so the spine surgeon will most likely kill or at least severely hurt our LVAD patient. So you see, we tell our patients, before any kind of medical examination or procedure, check with us. I advise you as well, dear reader, to always inform your VAD coordinator about planned invasive medical tests or procedures, especially if they are to be done in another hospital!

Back to the sleepless in Belgium, for him it was a given that the LVAD was keeping him from his sleep. "Do you hear the device?" "No." "Do you feel something in your chest maybe?" "No." For months we, a whole bunch of neurologists, sleep experts, everyone, looked into this sleeping problem, only to find nothing. Guess what? After one year the sleeping issue was over, without any medication or therapy. I still believe that he was somewhat afraid when he initially got his LVAD (although he never admitted it) and that he needed time to see that he could in fact live with this device. Once he acknowledged this, his sleepless nights were gone.

It is a common comment of patients, the fear of your life being dependent on a machine. It is a fear we can only try to imagine and have to take seriously. We can inform our patients about how much safer the devices have become over the years and point out the small number of true technical failures. But it is the same with a fear of flying. When you have it, you don't care how much safer planes are today as compared to the early days of flying and how small the risk of a crash is.

For me personally, the biggest fear would not be a technical failure of the pump, but a major stroke. A stroke can also kill you or cause disability for life, and it is far more frequent than a technical failure. Do you still remember Lucas, the young father who needed an LVAD to bring his pulmonary resistances down before he could be transplanted? Well, Lucas was on the LVAD for eight months when he had a minor stroke. He suddenly lost part of his sight, and although it recovered, the CT scan clearly showed a small ischemic zone in his brain. Lucas luckily didn't have any further issues with his LVAD and was transplanted later on. But not everyone is that lucky.

We lost one of our long-term LVAD patients to an unexpected and massive brain hemorrhage. He was first implanted with a second-generation LVAD. After six years, there was a clot inside the pump. He was a DT (destination therapy) patient in good physical health at that time. So he had an LVAD replacement and received a shiny, new third-generation device and a new aortic valve, as the old aortic valve was calcified and leaking moderately. When our head nurse retired five years later, he came and played a song he had written for her on his guitar. Yes he was a gifted musician. But one week after this last performance, we received a phone call from a nearby hospital. He was admitted there with a massive cerebral bleed, completely unresponsive. The only thing we could tell them was how to stop the pump . . .

Another patient we got to know in this book was Jan, the construction worker. Last time we met him, he had just left the hospital and was picking up medications at the pharmacy. Now, a few years later, Jan is not doing so well. He never fully recovered from the massive myocardial infarction he had. He had to stop working in construction and now has a desk job. Initially, it was not his cup of tea, but he managed to settle in there. He also gave up smoking, as well as alcohol and unhealthy food, but still to this day, he doesn't see any benefits of these conscious lifestyle choices.

Despite the perseverance of a healthy lifestyle, Jan has to be honest: it is not improving his health as if by a stroke of a magic wand. Worse yet, he feels that this is not really a life worth living anymore. He cannot stroll the streets anymore. Ten steps make him huff and puff just like a runner at the end of a marathon. This alarming trend hasn't gone unnoticed by his physicians. They know that Jan is not getting better. He is a good guy, and he's still quite young. Sadly, the unfortunate reality is that he's currently standing with one foot in the grave.

They informed Jan that he might need a new heart, but due to the long waiting lists and his worsening condition, he will need to rely on the active assistance of an LVAD. Later on, Jan received an LVAD in the BTD (bridge to decision) scenario. Six months after the implantation, no contraindications for a spot on the transplant waiting list were found—except for one, Jan himself. You see, Jan feels quite jittery, and the prospect of a second operation sounds a bit daunting, to say the least. Jan has read about transplants and spoken to the experts by experience, and as of today, he has come to the conclusion that for him, DT (destination therapy) is probably the best choice.

What do you think? What do I think? Well, again, as stipulated already a dozen times on the pages of this book: *every patient and every case are unique*. It truly is. For Jan, the team agreed that refraining from a transplantation was a good option. In other cases, we might think differently, and be assured, we will communicate this to you and explain our reasoning behind it. If you wonder if Jan made the right choice?

Well, he has had his LVAD now for seven years, we see him once a year, and he is happy. What would have happened if we had transplanted him? The truth is nobody knows. He might have been as happy as now, maybe even happier. Or maybe he would not even be here with us to tell his story.

This is one of the great struggles in surgery. Every procedure has a risk. On the other hand, doing nothing also has a risk. Oftentimes in cardiac surgery, doing nothing will result in a very high risk of dying. In these cases, choosing surgery is easy. But what if you do the operation for improved quality of life? If you do nothing in those cases, you will probably live another year or two (or three or more), but with heart failure symptoms. Still, the surgery in itself has a risk of fatality. Although small, the risk is there. To make these decisions, we physicians have to give our patients the correct information and listen to their needs and concerns. It is, after all, their life that is at stake. I'm proud that medicine has come this far. The times where a professor decided what needed to be done for a specific patient, regardless of the patient's opinion, are far behind us. A partnership with our patients working together to achieve the best outcome is our philosophy now.

Someone who didn't really have a choice was Peter, the young student with a nasty case of myocarditis. He needed the LVAD because he simply didn't have a functioning heart anymore. Peter was on the LVAD for eight months when a new heart arrived for him. Now he is back at college, studying again and going out for a drink from time to time, this time rocking a thick winter jacket.

As we have caught up with all our friends, now it's time to dive into the future! The next chapter will be pure science fiction and look at the future of heart pumps. This will be truly fascinating.

CHAPTER 9

THE FUTURE OF HEART PUMPS

MEDICAL SCIENCE IS A VERY INTERESTING DISCIPLINE, simply because it's always plowing ahead, expanding the boundaries of possibilities. As we go through this chapter, we will shine a light on new trends in the mechanical assistance of failing hearts. What does an ideal heart pump look like? What are the properties and physical boundaries to make this a reality? As we go ahead chewing on these important questions, let me assure you that the future of heart pumps is quite optimistic and somewhat rosy indeed. When it comes to treating the very late stages of heart failure, the steel heart has shown its potential as a valid therapy. I have no doubts that it will continue to do so for many years into the future.

Will the heart pump ever become a sort of a magic bullet against heart failure? Or will we eventually use a heart from a pig as an off-the-shelf, always available donor heart? Someday, these questions will be answered by brave doctors and engineers—landing them a place on the pages of medical history. For now, it's perfectly fine to daydream about these possibilities, however we always remain hungry for improvement.

What do you think of when you hear the word *modernization*? Most people associate this with making devices smaller, cleaner, smarter, and much more powerful. The same is happening in the world of long-term heart pumps. I'm happy to report that as time passes, we are amazed to see new improvements and space-age tech being developed and tested.

Let's start with the dimensions of our heart pump. Compared to the previous generation, the new designs are much more compact. After all, these first legacy heart pumps were simply too large to fit inside a patient's body. With time the pumps became small enough to be implanted into the patient's abdomen and subsequently even neatly nested inside the pericardium that surrounds the heart itself. What about reducing the size even more? What would be the maximum physical limit to the size of the perfect heart pump?

In the past, engineers came up with even smaller designs than what we currently use. Unfortunately, due to several factors that increase the risk of complications, we opted to stay away from these units. Subsequently, we gave up on further development altogether. The risks were just too high, and we cannot allow ourselves to subject our patients to such a high degree of questionable reliability and high risks.

The million-dollar question today is, "How small do we need a heart pump to be?" Remember, our mission is to attach the LVAD directly to the tip of the patient's heart (the apex) inside the pericardium (the layer of tissue that surrounds our heart). As you now know, we are working inside the very tight dimensions of the pericardium. Nature has ensured that there's simply no free space for any redundant or foreign material inside the confines of this pericardium. As we are implanting our heart pump, we need to make an incision into the pericardium in order to accommodate the steel heart. In an ideal situation, we would like to work with a thinner-shaped heart pump instead of a wider one. Why?

As the remodeling process of heart failure does its "dirty" job, it dilates the left ventricle, and the pericardium stretches along with it. So, at the tip of our heart (at the apex of the left ventricle), we have 5 to 6 cm of wiggle room to the sides that's ideal for our heart pump implantation. A pump that's only 2 cm tall and 6 cm wide simply works much better than one that is 4 cm high and 4 cm wide. As we are pondering the dimensions of the ideal pump designs, we always have to account for those inevitable laws of physics. As we move away from the heart pump's rotor, we enter a special outflow tube that leads to the aorta. Over the years, we have learned that the minimal diameter of this tube cannot be smaller than 1 cm. Anything lower would cause too much drag and resistance to the blood flow.

This is why it is safe to say that the smallest and most compact pump design would never be thinner than 1 cm. For us surgeons, this would be music to our ears. Such a design would greatly reduce the complexity of implantation surgery and allow our patients to recover much faster. As an added side effect, these heart pumps would also be able to help children and people with an overall smaller anatomy. As we daydream further, let's think about the power output of such a hypothetical heart pump. By now you already know that most heart pumps are fully capable of circulating a whopping five liters of blood every minute. This corresponds with the blood flow of an average adult who's not performing any demanding physical activity.

In optimal conditions, we can speed things up and allow a modern heart pump to circulate up to eight liters per minute when needed. This can only be achieved when we can ensure an ample (and quick) delivery of blood flow to the heart pump every step of the way. In medical terms, that would mean having a proper working right ventricle function as well as low lung resistance. If these conditions are not met, the left ventricle won't be properly filled with blood, and the heart pump will literally suck it dry. As you remember from previous chapters, a suction alarm will quickly remind our patient when this scenario occurs in practice.

To an untrained eye, it would seem that going from five to eight liters (an increase of 60 percent in blood flow) would already be an amazing achievement. Sadly, this is nowhere near enough. You see, a healthy, athletic human heart is capable of cranking out up to twenty-five liters per minute as you huff and puff during heavy physical performance. Most of our patients with a steel heart would never need such earth-shattering peak performance blood flow numbers. When it comes to younger patients, their exercise capacity remains limited despite a perfectly working heart pump assisting them along the way.

Now, we already told you that speeding up current heart pumps won't give our patients any significant athletic boost, but we can always be optimistic for the future. As we gain more knowledge and experience, we will design and build smarter heart pumps that one day will allow our patients to run marathons. That must be our goal, and though probably hard to achieve, we like to aim high. At the moment, we are pretty much limited to eight liters of blood flow per minute.

Personally, I believe that a heart pump capable of up to fifteen liters per minute definitely deserves its place under the sun. This increased blood flow is not only fantastic for physical exercises, but it would also greatly benefit patients in other ways—when we are ill or when we hit a high fever, our cardiac output needs to increase just to keep our blood pressure steady. I'm very excited to see this technology being developed (and used) during our lifetime.

When it comes to innovation, efficiency is on everyone's lips. Our phones, cars, and other appliances are becoming faster and much smarter when it comes to energy usage. We expect new models and new designs to last longer and go much further than before. Let's examine the heart pump's energy efficiency.

If in the past, a battery could provide just six hours of use. Today, we are breaking the boundaries of twelve or even sixteen hours with ease. This is possible due to innovative pump design and improvement of battery technology. Can we expect the next generation of heart pumps to be even more energy efficient? Definitely—yet it's important to mention that today we have already reached a quite well-manageable battery life for our patients. But as we dream on, twenty-four hours of stress-free mobility with even lighter and smaller batteries would be nice.

To put this into perspective, you could then safely jump on an airplane and travel from one continent to another without any headache or "charging stress" as your steel heart is leisurely buzzing every single second of your trip. That being said, let's always remember to take a spare battery with us just in case (you never know what can happen).

Yes, with time the batteries will become even more compact, allowing for greater comfort and ease of use for our patients. Having access to outside power sources (like a portable solar panel for example) and a few spare batteries, we would even be able to stretch this hassle-free period to a few days. With time, this will eliminate the so-called charging stress that's so common among drivers of electric vehicles (and coincidently among heart pump patients as well).

As good as things may be today, we are still only relatively happy with the performance of the current heart pump models. Let's keep in mind that the Achilles' heel is still the exposed driveline that exits the patient's abdomen. Our ideal scenario is to see a complete system (heart pump, control unit, and battery) that we can fully implant into the patient's body—eliminating the risk of driveline infections as a result. Of course, this is easier said than done. You see, by eliminating one problem (exposed driveline), we inevitably create a plethora of potentially new problems that need addressing.

We have already learned to make an amazingly reliable heart pump. As it performs flawlessly for many years, it will demand a monstrous amount of energy that needs to be stored inside and delivered by a battery. During normal operation, an LVAD uses a small 5 W of energy. So over ten years this would add up to almost half a megawatt of energy. Such a battery that is small enough to fit inside your body simply doesn't exist. Now you have an understanding of what we're dealing with today. Technology simply hasn't caught up with us yet. Aside from a miniature nuclear reactor, we don't have access to that kind of battery technology.

Yes, you heard it correctly—nuclear! This is not a joke. In the 1960s, doctors and engineers conducted research into implantable miniature nuclear reactors. This radical idea was eventually shelved due to those pesky laws of physics. You see, aside from the obvious dangers of radiation, a potential micro-reactor has a risk of overheating, and frankly, it's just too bulky to be considered implantable. In medicine, this simply doesn't work. Today we can only find RTGs (*radioisotope thermo-electric generators*) in many remote places around the world. Usually these types of (rather bulky) power sources work nonstop for many decades, providing power to unmanned lighthouses, radio communication stations, and even deep-space exploration probes.

For the past few decades, we have been exploring the possibilities of transcutaneous energy transfer (TET). Pioneered by Nikola Tesla, this amazing wireless transmission of energy is called *induction charging*. We see this in our handheld devices such as smartphones and tablets. The basic principle is quite simple: two copper coils (one hidden inside a charger and another one inside the battery pack) transmit energy from the charger to the battery. During the entire process, energy "hovers" across one coil to another, bypassing air or other materials.

Let's think out loud for a second. What if we make the charging coil implantable? We would immediately do away with the highest risk of infection (an exposed driveline) and allow our patient to wirelessly provide power to their heart pump. Yes, this is an amazing idea. However, we quickly run into a dilemma: Will we be transferring power to the heart pump directly? Or will we use it to power an implantable battery pack? As you may already imagine, the best solution would be to power the heart pump directly.

Think about it for a second. We want nothing more than to avoid the need for a battery altogether—just imagine having to undergo surgical procedures just to replace the battery every time it has degraded. Besides, the battery can quickly become hot during charging, and this is something we want to avoid at all costs.

On the other hand, if the patient doesn't have a battery powering the heart pump, the TET system would require a constant presence of the charging coil on the patient's body. In other words, a patient would need to permanently wear a battery pack and an induction coil. Out with the annoying driveline, in with a new system that needs to be carried around at all times. Now imagine if the two coils were not aligned perfectly—the heart pump would simply stop working. As you can see, designing such a perfect system is quite a tough nut to crack.

But the minds of engineers never rest, and now a kind of piercing is being tested as a TET system. One ring under your skin, the second pierced right through the center of the internal ring. This system is quite small, and as the rings are pierced together, there is no risk of decoupling between them. Definitely technology that I keep an eye on!

But as I allow myself to daydream about sci-fi technology, I would personally (and professionally) choose a system with a highly efficient and durable implantable battery that would outlast five years of flawless operation and that guarantees a twenty-four-hour autonomy to the patient. In practice, the patient would charge that battery with a TET system during the night, while during the day they could disconnect the charging coil and head out into the world to live a normal life (without the need for external battery packs or other paraphernalia). I dream of the day that I will finally be able to work with such a system, allowing our patients the ultimate freedom and mobility.

What about the control unit, you may ask? I'm glad you brought this up. Yes, the control unit definitely needs to become smaller, tougher, and implantable. It needs to be smarter, too—equipped with the ability to send alarms to an external device such as your phone or smartwatch. You may not know this, but wireless communication systems for such vital devices (remember we are talking about life-and-death scenarios) have to conform to strict norms and regulations. Again, developing such a controller is easier said than done.

Would such a totally implantable system with fancy TET coils and batteries be the perfect solution for everyone?

Imagine that you happen to find yourself in a bridge to transplant (BTT) scenario. Would you actually want an entire implantable system inside your body? After all, all the devices that are implanted will eventually need to be removed during the transplant procedure. Today, with just a pump and a driveline, this can already be quite a challenging surgical procedure. Imagine that you also need to dig out a TET coil, controller, and battery pack during that surgery! We would not like to see our patients suffer this kind of trauma. What about only explanting the heart and the heart pump during the transplantation and leaving all the rest inside? This, unfortunately, is also a bad idea. You see, as the patient is under the required doses of immunosuppressive medications (these are needed to prevent your body from rejecting a donor heart), the consequences of even a minor infection can become life-threatening. The decommissioned controller, battery, and coil inside your body would become hot spots for infection.

Personally, I can already see a future where we will have several solutions that will suit the needs of different patients.

For example, patients who have a high chance of accepting a donor heart (or perhaps someone who has a high chance of recovering their natural heart function in its entirety) would be outfitted with a classic LVAD system with a driveline that exits the abdomen.

Or they could benefit from having a catheter-mounted pump that sits only inside the blood vessels. This even means that the surgery to do the heart transplant would be their first surgery. This might not seem important, but after every operation, adhesions form inside the operated area. As you do surgery again in the same region, the tissues don't separate nicely but stick together, like they are glued. This increases the risks of bleeding and complications. So, if we could avoid having to go inside your chest twice for surgery, we would definitely do so.

These catheter-mounted pumps will probably play a greater role in the future. The implantation procedure is fast and straightforward without having to open the chest. If such pumps would allow for two to three years of uninterrupted performance, it would be more than enough to allow the patient to recover their complete heart function (or wait for a donor heart to become available). Today these catheter-mounted pumps are only used for a few weeks to months at most, but catheter-mounted pumps that would allow support for months to a year are being developed as we speak.

Everything changes when we are dealing with a patient who doesn't meet the criteria for a heart transplantation. We are, of course, speaking about the destination therapy (DT) scenario here. In this case we can definitely work with a fully implantable system, and the only risk is replacing partially defective components as the years of living without a heartbeat go by. Over the whole history of heart pumps, we have seen just one fully implantable system, called the Lionheart.

As we explore the future of heart pumps, we need to focus on developing smarter pumps. What do we mean by smarter? You already know that sometimes an inlet cannula of the LVAD can grab the inner lining of the ventricle and become stuck to it. Today's pumps immediately decrease their speed when this happens to release the ventricular wall. A smart LVAD, on the other hand, would not only take action to let go of the inner lining of the ventricle but would also predict when such a suction event would be likely to happen. Now this is innovation!

As we speak, engineers and doctors are conducting research into doing just that—building smarter heart pumps that would predict the risk of suction events. The heart pump would need just a few seconds to adjust itself in order to prevent such an event from occurring. This system requires sensors and other nifty tech to work properly. Again, this presents us with other important hurdles that we need to address. As you now know, our blood doesn't like rubbing shoulders with foreign material such as sensors. Our body is quite good at recognizing and rejecting anything that doesn't belong. In fact, our body would go to extreme lengths to grow a layer of tissue over anything it dislikes, just to prevent this nasty intruder from damaging the sanctity of our biological perfection.

Nowhere can this be seen better than inside the outflow graft that runs from the LVAD to our aorta. With time, our body starts to grow a layer of tissue over the graft simply because it sees this graft as a foreign object. This layer of tissue transforms the graft into an extension of our own blood vessels. Not only is this incredibly cool, but it also prevents blood clots from forming inside the tube. We cannot stop at being in awe of the capabilities of the human body.

Now what do you think would happen to sophisticated sensors peppered throughout the steel heart? Such sensors (that measure our blood flow and pressure) would inevitably be seen as foreign objects in dire need of a new layer of tissue—rendering their readings unreliable (or even completely useless) over time. All of this takes place inside our body without easy access for potential replacement. After all, our mission is to ensure many years of flawless reliability. As of today, we see a few prototype sensors that can be connected to the heart pump and feed us reliable data for years, but sadly they aren't clinically available just yet. What about the pump itself?

Yes, we can make the steel heart smarter and let the device adapt itself to the needs of the body that it serves. Today's heart pumps are always buzzing at the same speed (day and night). During the night, the speed can probably be lower, while during the day it may need to increase to accommodate the needs of an active lifestyle. As you remember, simply tinkering with the speed of the heart pump won't lead to a sizable increase in the physical performance of our patients. Perhaps in the future we can use a smarter way of handling these speed increases. For example, the speed could increase only during one part of the heart cycle. Or maybe the pump can speed up during periods of rising pressure inside the left ventricle.

In some (rare) cases we see our LVAD patients recover their natural heart function. A smarter heart pump would be able to detect this and naturally modify the assistance to the left ventricle. This way we would even be able to train a patient's natural heart to work fully by itself during certain periods of time. As technology evolves, these dreams will one day become reality. For now, we need to bow our heads over a small mountain of crucial research.

We need better sensors. We need to learn about the marriage between our biological heart and the steel heart, and most of all, we need to learn about all the mechanisms that cause heart failure. All the new knowledge and discoveries will inevitably translate into new software that will drive better and smarter LVADs. As of today, we can only do so much research. Consider that conducting research into rare illnesses and therapies is quite difficult and cumbersome. We simply don't have enough data (or sometimes data collecting just takes a long time). This is why every tiny morsel of research and heart pump development is an entirely global effort. Why do you think you're reading this book in English?

Today there are specialists all over the world bowing their heads and bundling their efforts to collect data and conduct vital research. People from Europe, Asia, the Americas, and many other countries are chipping in and offering their time, knowledge, and research for the greater good of humanity. This allows us to work much faster and more effectively than ever before. Some examples of these collaborations are the ISMCS (International Society of Mechanical Circulatory Support) or the IMACS (ISHLT Mechanically Assisted Circulatory Support) registry. This collaboration allows us to build and expand an impressive collection of data from European, American, and Asian databases.

What will all these future innovations look like? As we covered the history of the heart pumps, we saw that we started out with pulsatile designs, moving on to rotor-equipped pumps (of the second-generation) and eventually ending up with the much more reliable magnetic heart pumps of the third-generation we know and love today. Someday these designs will be retired to the pages of medical history books. Today, we are already experimenting with propelling blood using vibrating membranes (that work much like a fish tail). I'm extremely excited to see what the brilliant minds will come up with during our lifetime. Medical innovation never sleeps and is never satisfied with (already impressive) past achievements, as perfection is not yet reached.

CHAPTER 10

END OF LIFE WITH A HEART PUMP

ONE OF THE MOST COMMON QUESTIONS PATIENTS AND caretakers ask is, "Can you die with a heart pump?" After all, the steel heart takes over the heart's function. You can only die once your heart fully stops, right? Will the heart pump keep working in this scenario? Unfortunately, it's not all that simple. Let's take some time to unpack everything and bring closure to these important questions.

The presumption of death due to the heart ceasing its function is completely wrong. Nevertheless, this definition has been circulating inside our collective mindset (and community) for quite a long time. And for a long time, the definition was spot on to define death. In the mid-twentieth century, death was defined by the cessation of breathing and pulse. So, in fact, every ECMO patient would be dead by that definition. They don't breathe because the ECMO does it for them, and their blood pressure shows no pulsatility. Needless to say, medical progression has been pushing not only the boundaries of actual death (like a deep hypothermic circulatory arrest, for example) but also the legal definition of death. Therefore, the medical field moved on to define other criteria for death, and the concept of brain death was added. Being brain-dead means that there is such massive and irreversible brain damage that it is no longer compatible with life.

Naturally, this also creates problems of acceptance of the legal definition of death. Some think it goes too far, and I'm sure that at some point you have heard in the media about legal trials on this topic. In this book, I don't want to make statements about these definitions, but the fact that the definition of death is seen as broader than just cessation of pulse and breathing is important to highlight here. When you read this book, please realize again that we are referring here to a Belgian situation. Laws and practices might be different in your home country. An important given in any definition of death is its irreversibility. Death has to be irreversible! This is logical, because if it is reversible, then treat the damn patient!

If we translate this to our patients with a heart pump, does this mean that they can only die of brain death? The answer is no. Why? Let's find out!

The steel heart performs a supporting function—it assists the hard work of our left ventricle and sends pressurized blood to our aorta (and subsequently to other arteries). In order to do it properly, blood needs to be present in the left ventricle. If this is not the case (for example, due to increased lung resistance or right heart failure), the heart pump will simply receive no blood at all. The left ventricle will be sucked dry, and the pressure inside the arteries will drop. In this scenario, the patient will first lose consciousness and (if this dire situation continues) eventually pass away due to insufficient blood flow.

On the other hand, even with a perfectly functioning heart (and low lung resistance), it is in fact possible to see a patient pass away, for example, due to massive bleeding. This scenario can happen during an intestinal bleeding event. Sometimes massive bleeding can occur inside the brain. In other cases blood clots can start blocking the arteries to our brains and eventually cause irreversible brain damage—triggering a fatal chain of events. In short, a patient with a steel heart doesn't automatically become immune to the natural laws of life and death, and they are just as vulnerable as any of us.

There are some patients that deserve a special mention—people who suffer from irregular heart rhythms. You may not know this, but many patients who suffer from long-term heart failure (and who currently live with a steel heart) are equipped with an internal defibrillator. This tiny device resembles a normal pacemaker, and it's constantly monitoring the heart rhythm. Every time the device notices a life-threatening heart rhythm, it will immediately administer an electric shock. This happens only when the heart rhythm is too fast or too divergent from a normal, steady pace. After all, during these events the heart cannot function to its fullest capacity, and the blood flow throughout the body is severely impacted. How bad can it get?

As the blood pressure drops due to the irregular heart rhythm, the patient can faint and eventually even die. In this situation, the small "internal defibrillator" will fire off an electric shock and try to kickstart the restless heart. This electric shock is only administered a few seconds after the irregular rhythm has started. You see, quite often, the irregular heart rhythm can subside on its own, and it's quite prudent to wait even a few seconds before the device moves on to drastic measures. Another advantage of waiting a few seconds before unleashing the electric hell is that the patient slips into a state of unconsciousness.

Believe me, this is a definite benefit—being kicked by an "electric mule" in a conscious state is a serious traumatic event indeed.

Let's imagine that our patient lives with a steel heart and their lung resistance is nice and low. If this patient is hijacked by an irregular heart rhythm event, you can already imagine what will happen—the blood pressure will not fall, simply because the blood pump is assisting the heart every step of the way.

Most patients with a heart pump who find themselves in this exact situation will feel "something odd," but in no way will they even begin to lose consciousness or arrive at a fatal outcome. Trust me when I say it, but this would be the worst place to be in, as the electric mule thinks that you are currently fainting and proceeds to resuscitate your heart with high voltage. This is also the reason why we often deactivate the internal defibrillator as the patient with irregular heart rhythm is outfitted with a brand-new steel heart.

Since we mention resuscitation, it's quite important to understand this procedure, as it also applies to our steel heart patients. As you now know, these patients can have a total lack of a noticeable heartbeat in their peripheral arteries. To say that this can be confusing is an understatement. Imagine that our patient simply fainted and lost consciousness. The lack of a palpable heartbeat can already be a trigger for full-on resuscitation. Unfortunately, this can happen in real life.

So first of all, it is important to realize that not every person who suddenly loses consciousness and collapses is having a cardiac arrest. There are many reasons why this can happen while the heart simply keeps on beating as usual. Sometimes it can be epileptic seizures, maybe a stroke or hypoglycemia (lack of glucose in the bloodstream). How can we handle these scenarios and help our patients to the best of our ability? We'll still follow the ABCs of a classic resuscitation procedure. If you're curious, *A* is for *airways*, *B* is for *breathing*, and *C* is for *circulation*. Ready?

Step 1. Are the airways free? When there are no obstructions inside the airways, we can safely proceed to B.

Step 2. Is the patient spontaneously breathing or not? Oxygen is the highest priority! Once this step is covered, we can safely move on.

Step 3. Does the patient have normal blood circulation? This is where things get tricky! Our patient has a heart pump, and the pulse can only be measured with highly specialized equipment that lives within the confines of hospital walls. What now?

In all normal situations, we can check the patient's pulse by feeling the arteries around the neck or groin. In these places, our major arteries are close to the skin surface and can be easily located to check for the presence of a healthy pulse. Right now we don't feel a pulse and mistakenly conclude that the patient needs a heart massage technique to regain normal heart function. However, patients with a steel heart don't have a pulse, and yet there might be ample blood circulating around the body and performing all the necessary functions for sustaining life. How can we rule out the possibility of mistakenly giving a steel heart patient an unnecessary heart massage?

First, we start with a thorough check of the patient. You already know about the temperamental control unit. Initially, the controller notices that the heart pump is not generating the needed blood flow. As the blood flow drops to critical levels, the controller will send out a screeching alarm sound to notify the patient (and bystanders) that something serious is happening. Imagine that the patient is lying unconscious, and you don't hear any alarms from the control unit. This means the circulation is there and the steel heart is buzzing away at its leisure (the *C* of the ABCs is perfectly normal).

Next, we need to consult the controller to have a rough estimate of how much blood is flowing through the body of our patient every minute. I remember vividly when patients were resuscitated in the emergency room while their blood flow measured by the controller was more than 4 L per minute. Needless to say, I almost had to fight the other doctors just to persuade them to stop the heart massage. As you remember, our instinct is to keep the heart massage going until we feel a strong pulse. It's not always easy to be completely sure that the patient's circulation is functioning as it should. When a patient with a heart pump is unconscious it usually means that there is a serious problem. Even if it is not a cardiac arrest, the blood flow still may be affected and lower than normal. It goes without saying that will trigger a whole series of various controller alarms, and blood flow data shown on the controller screen will be lower than usual. How can we know that there's ample blood circulation?

Enter capillary refill! Capillaries are tiny blood vessels spread out across every square centimeter of our body. All these capillaries need blood flow just like any of our major arteries do. This is where capillary refill comes in. Instead of explaining it, let's just see it in action! Use your left index finger to push on the top of your right index finger. You'll quickly notice that the skin under the nail of your right index finger immediately turns white. Fascinating to see, isn't it?

Currently you're using your finger to squeeze the blood out of your tiny capillaries. No blood—no healthy pink hue in the skin! As you remove the pressure that your left index finger is exerting, you'll see the skin under the nail of your right index finger turn pink again. Now you know how capillary refill works, let's examine what happens when there's not enough blood circulation. You can already predict the outcome—it will take much longer to see the fingernail change color from white to pink. Even when you're not feeling a pulse from a patient with a steel heart, it will take just two seconds to see the capillary refill in action (playing out under the fingernail of the patient). Anything longer than two seconds can mean only one thing—not enough blood flow! This is when we immediately need to start the heart massage.

Here's another top tip when you are helping an unconscious heart pump patient: look at the control unit. The phone number of the hospital where the heart pump was implanted will be mentioned there. If the patient is experiencing a serious episode, it's always a good idea to call this number immediately. The VAD coordinator (just like guardian angels) will provide you with all the relevant information that will greatly help your resuscitation efforts. They can also provide you with helpful tips on how to suppress the control unit alarms and guide you through the intricacies of the control unit's settings.

If our patient enters the emergency room of the nearest hospital, any standard resuscitation procedure simply won't work. Any patient equipped with a heart pump requires a bespoke approach. First of all, many ER units will have specialized equipment to assist with the resuscitation efforts. This heart massage machine is genius in its consistency and effectiveness. Imagine a bow-shaped structure that holds a large pounder (it looks a bit like a large plunger). The entire construction is installed just above the patient's chest. This machine can now perform the heart massage and allow the doctors the freedom and maneuverability to help the patient further. Another advantage of these special machines is the consistent quality of chest compressions—every single time, the pounder will compress the patient's chest with the same speed and force. Sadly, the same cannot be said when this procedure is executed by humans (who find themselves in quite a stressful situation or get tired after a while).

This space-age machine has helped doctors save countless lives. What about our heart pump patients? Here's where things get tricky again. We prefer not to use this machine! You see, the powerful compressions of the resuscitation machine can damage the heart by compressing the soft and quite fragile heart muscle against the rigid inflow cannula and, in the worst case, even rip the heart pump off the left ventricle entirely. If this happens, we won't be able to save our patient, no matter how hard we try.

As the heart pump technology evolves and improves, we are happy to report that our patients are living much longer and much more fulfilling lives. Yet, sometimes DT (destination therapy) patients do ask to explore the possibility of euthanasia. In the past few years, we have seen this trend increase. The heart pump is not the culprit in these scenarios. Today we are seeing a change in the patient's mentality, whereby people want to have full control over the precise moment when they close their fulfilled life and step through the tunnel of light.

The legal requirements regarding euthanasia apply to every individual, including our heart pump patients. In practice, the entire procedure looks quite different. The VAD coordinator will have to stop the LVAD during this process. There are ongoing discussions about whether stopping the LVAD should be seen as euthanasia or as a cessation of a therapy. Again, as the definition of death, this is a legal minefield, and we will not go further into this discussion in this book. Please do consider that every country will have different regulations on this topic.

When a patient's steel heart has completed its final rotation, the soul can finally exit the biological suit that served it for so many years. What happens to the heart pump in this case? Is it left inside the patient's body? When a body is cremated, pacemakers are always removed because they can explode. The heart pump doesn't have internal batteries (yet) and therefore can simply be left inside the patient's body.

EPILOGUE

I TRULY HOPE YOU HAD AS MUCH PLEASURE READING this book as I had writing it. I hope it gave you a better understanding of what artificial heart pumps are and how we use them in our daily practice. This book is meant in the first place for LVAD patients and their loved ones. Living with an LVAD or seeing a loved one connected to a short-term assist device in the ICU is a shock. This book might help you better understand why it was needed and what the future may hold. Also, caregivers who happen to come along a patient with an LVAD might find some background here. I do realize that this high-tech and still quite rare treatment option for heart failure patients can be new even to them.

Let's not forget that when medical science and technology meet, wonderful things can happen. Such as the invention of mechanical hearts. So last, this book is for everyone who loves to learn about medicine and it's cutting-edge inventions!

So, dear reader, my last advice to you:

Perhaps today you're a healthy young person in the prime of your life. As you close this book, I want to ask you to think about how our modern lifestyle constantly conspires to make us as passive and lazy as possible. The simple truth (that you already know from your childhood) is that we are meant to be active. The saying, "When you rest, you rust," applies to every muscle fiber of your body. Hopefully this book was a wake-up call that you were subconsciously seeking all this time. I'm absolutely sure that you will use this knowledge to your best advantage.

Or maybe you already carry the burden of a heart condition. In that case keep fighting that awful disease and know that you're not alone.

Doctors, engineers, nurses, and countless other healthcare practitioners are by your side. And remember, thanks to medical science, there is literally a way to give yourself a second chance. Now you know how it all works.

And finally:

As a long-time medical professional, I would like to finish by saying that for as long as you live, I hope we never have to see each other in the hospital!

END

www.ingramcontent.com/pod-product-compliance
Lightning Source LLC
Chambersburg PA
CBHW062131020426
42335CB00013B/1180